An Easier
Childbirth

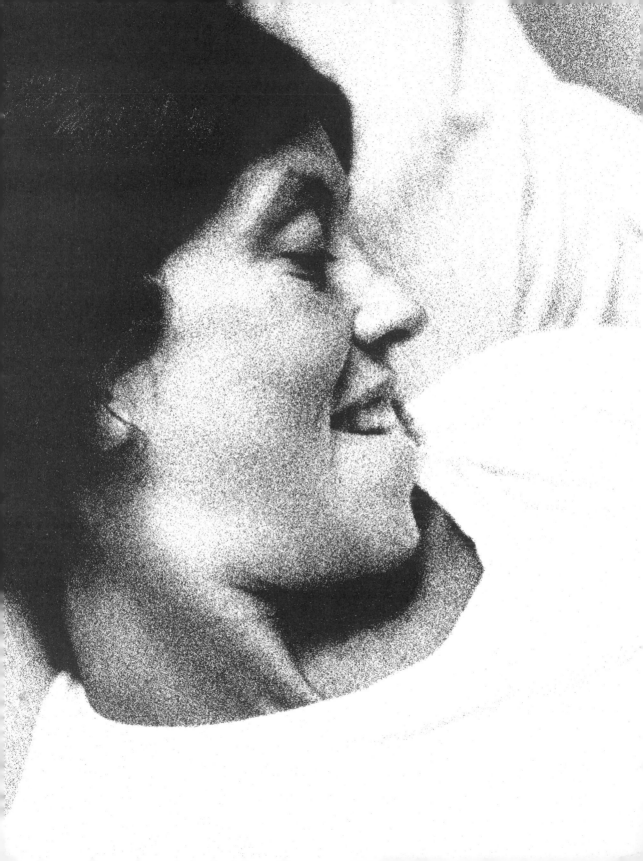

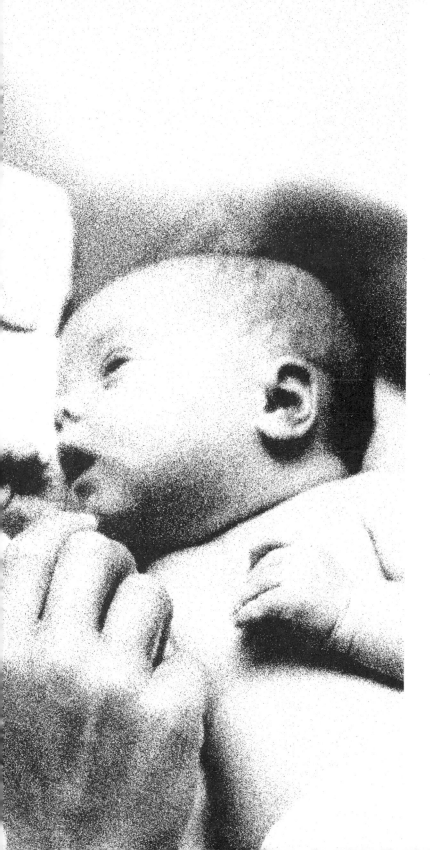

An Easier
Childbirth

*A Mother's Workbook
for Health
and Emotional
Well-Being
during Pregnancy
and Delivery*

Gayle Peterson, Ph.D.

Foreword by Sheila Kitzinger

JEREMY P. TARCHER, INC.
Los Angeles

ALSO BY GAYLE PETERSON

Birthing Normally

Cesarean Birth: Risk and Culture
(WITH LEWIS MEHL)

*A Chance to Live: Children's Poems
for Peace in a Nuclear Age*
(COEDITED WITH YING LEE KELLEY)

Pregnancy as Healing
(WITH LEWIS MEHL)

Library of Congress Cataloging-in-Publication Data

Peterson, Gayle H.
    An easier childbirth : a mother's workbook for health and
emotional well-being during pregnancy and delivery / Gayle Peterson.
        p.   cm.
    Includes bibliographical references and index.
    ISBN 0-87477-665-1
    1. Pregnancy—Popular works.   2. Childbirth—Popular works.
    I. Title.
RG525.P434   1991   91-24383
    618.2'4—dc20   CIP

Jeremy P. Tarcher, Inc.
5858 Wilshire Blvd., Suite 200
Los Angeles, CA 90036

Distributed by St. Martin's Press, New York

Design by Susan Shankin
Interior photography by Harriette Hartigan

Manufactured in the United States of America
10 9 8 7 6 5 4 3 2 1

First Edition

This book is dedicated
to my husband,
Stuart Gold,
who taught me
the meaning of family.

CONTENTS

ACKNOWLEDGMENTS

I WOULD LIKE TO acknowledge the following people for their support and contributions. My deepest and heartfelt thanks to my editors, Andrea Stein and Mary Ellen Strote; my good friend and colleague Greg Bogart; Carol Brendsel, R.N.; Marianne Reidman at the Monterey Bay Aquarium for her expertise on sea mammals; Mary Davenport, M.D.; Paula Holtz, C.N.M.; Kate Bowland, C.N.M.; Jeri Zukoski, C.N.M.; Nora Swan-Foster, Judy Lazarus, Terri Ray, Stuart Gold, and, last but not least, my wonderful teenagers—Sorrel and Yarrow Madrona.

I also wish to express my deepest gratitude to all the women and families I worked with—for giving me the opportunity to learn from them.

FOREWORD

CHILDBIRTH IS AS MUCH about all that goes on in our minds as our bodies. It is the same with other physiological processes: sex, digestion, the way we move, our facial expressions, our physical gestures, and how we stand and walk.

Pain in childbirth, like any other kind of pain, is never merely a physical stimulus. It is interpreted by our minds. In the sixties when Lamaze training was introduced to the United States from France, its focus was on the eradication of pain by conditioned responses to contractions, and women who still had painful labors often felt that they had failed because the pain refused to go away.

In *The Complete Book of Pregnancy and Childbirth*, first published in 1980, I explored instead the concept of "pain with a purpose." I suggested that we should think about pain in a normal birth as qualitatively different from other kinds of pain. This may be difficult to accept for anyone who has not experienced the positive pain of uterine contractions, the dilating cervix, and the pressure of the baby's head as it slides down through the flexible passage of the birth canal and spreads wide the tissues of the vagina and perineum. Physical effort, for example when we run a race or climb a mountain, produces *functional* pain, the ache of muscles that are working hard. Gayle Peterson has developed this idea of psychological preparation for birth in order to enable a woman to handle "healthy pain," and to release the pain freely, without inhibitions.

In pregnancy it is important to think about pain and our attitudes toward it. Relaxing completely is only one way of dealing with pain. A woman in childbirth may want to move, to pound the floor, to squeeze a partner's hand, to moan or yell or hiss. There are auditory and kinesthetic ways of coping that are often frowned on because attendants think that the woman must be "out of control." Yet these can be just as useful as the more socially acceptable technique of patterned breathing, and each woman should be free to discover what works for her. Everything in the mind of a woman in childbirth is profoundly influenced by the social context in which birth takes place—the assumptions about what birth is, who should help, and what are appropriate ways of helping. The social system within which any woman gives birth validates certain kinds of knowledge, while other ways of knowing are considered irrelevant.

In an authoritarian, high-tech, hierarchical medical system, women's knowledge about themselves, about their own bodies and what they are feeling, is discredited. The only valid knowledge is that sanctioned by doctors. Women are expected to be the passive recipients of medical care. They are denied access to information and are not allowed to share in decision-making, except in a superficial and marginal way.

Women in childbirth are usually restricted to an institutional environment which, even when it has been made "homey" with hanging plants, a rocking chair, and a patchwork quilt, makes them feel that they must defer to the professionals in charge, whom they are conditioned to believe know more about them than they can possibly know themselves.

As a result, a woman in labor is forced to discount her own knowledge and her intense feelings. She struggles against her body to get the baby born instead of working with it, fights the pain instead of accepting and passing *through* it, and is trapped in conflict between the messages she is receiving from her body and the instructions she hears from her attendants.

We cannot solve these problems by childbirth education. Or at least, we cannot solve them if childbirth education is aimed only at pregnant women. There is urgent need for childbirth education for *doctors and nurses* so that, instead of superimposing a medical perception of birth, professional helpers listen to, learn from, and respect women's experiences. Only in this way shall we be able to humanize the culture of birth.

In these pages Gayle Peterson gets to the heart of the experience of childbirth. It is not just a question of "an easier birth," but of a woman's passion and striving, her longing and fulfilment, and the power of her body to bring new life into the world.

Sartre, in his book *Existentialism and Humanism* says: "Life is nothing until it is lived, but it is yours to make sense of, and the value of it is nothing else but the sense that you choose." Birth, too, is nothing until it is lived, and each of us has the opportunity to make sense of it according to our own deepest values.

Sheila Kitzinger

INTRODUCTION

WHEN I BECAME PREGNANT with my daughter in the spring of 1973, I was twenty-two years old. I had graduated recently from Indiana University with a degree in psychology, but had not given much thought to motherhood. The pregnancy was unplanned; if anyone had asked me before that whether I wanted to have children someday, I would have replied with a definite no. The responsibilities of parenthood brought up fear; they were not part of my life plan. Once I learned that I was six weeks pregnant, however, I was surprised by unexpected feelings of attachment to the unborn child. My husband's excitement about having a baby helped me decide to continue the pregnancy. I did not yet know the richness that this decision would bring to my future. Nor could I have imagined that I would look back on this period of pregnancy, childbirth, and new motherhood as a pivotal event of my life—the cornerstone of my professional, as well as personal, development.

Early in my pregnancy I decided to give birth at home. I had discovered that in most American hospitals, fathers and friends were banned from the delivery room, and babies were whisked away to the nursery as soon as they emerged. Women whose physicians were acquainted with the work of natural-childbirth advocates such as Dick-Read, Lamaze, and Bradley were sometimes able to arrange for more humane conditions. Women who did not prepare for a natural childbirth or who had complications in labor risked having an emotionally ungratifying delivery.

The medical community's unsatisfactory response to women's emotional needs during childbirth and women's growing desire to take charge of their health care had generated a grassroots home-birth movement. Many women turned to lay midwives, who provided the emotional sensitivity that was lacking in traditional hospital settings. The research that would ultimately promote changes in and arrangements for maternity wards, including alternative birthing rooms where families could stay together during and after the birth, had not yet been conducted. Ultimately, I would become one of the researchers who would support consumer demands for changes in hospital policy. But I chose to deliver my baby at home simply because I felt that separation from my husband and close women friends would have a negative effect on my labor. I wanted to be with my baby during the first hours of life. Even in my inexperience, I sensed that emotional variables could have an impact on my baby's birth.

I was fortunate to have received my prenatal care from lay midwives who prepared me for labor both physically and psychologically. Their gentle questions guided me to contemplation of this period of growth and change. My exploration of significant childhood memories and feelings helped me identify the kind of mother I wanted to be.

The midwives also encouraged their patients to learn from each other. We waited for our prenatal appointments in the living room of an old Victorian house, the home of my midwife, Kate. Mothers who had recently given birth shared their experiences with those of us who were pregnant, imparting realistic information about childbirth. Their birth stories helped me develop resources that I brought to my own labor. Although I had attended Lamaze preparation classes where I'd seen movies of women giving birth, none of these films had the impact of one uncensored audiotape that I was lucky enough to hear while I waited for my last prenatal appointment.

I will never forget Ann's playing the audiotape of herself in labor, while she waited for her postpartum visit. The sounds of her wailing during a contraction resounded throughout the waiting area, as she nursed her two-week-old baby. I listened to this woman's labor and at the same time watched her smile at her newborn. At once, both the reality of labor pain and the beauty of birth were communicated to me. The sounds of Ann's labor provided me with a type of body education that my childbirth classes had lacked and readied me to meet my own labor without fear.

My daughter's birth was a very moving experience for me. It was a natural childbirth, and I delivered her at home after eight hours of active labor, during which I felt the power of the life force traveling through me. That feeling came again with the birth of my son three years later. Both times I felt lucky to be a woman. I was able to meet, and enjoy, this experience only because I integrated the emotional work of this period of my life into my preparation for childbirth.

Wanting to share the richness of my own experience, I immersed myself in research on the safety of home delivery to see if my choice could be a viable one for other women. Lewis Mehl, M.D., Donald Creevy, M.D., Nancy Shaw, Ph.D., and I studied the outcomes of home births attended by Santa Cruz midwives in the early 1970s. Our initial research encouraged us to study prenatal care. This work led me to explore the way that emotional and psychological factors affect normal and healthy labors in any setting— home or hospital. Emotional factors proved second only to physical health and nutrition in importance for a normal labor and delivery.

During the past two decades, medical researchers have documented how a woman's emotional state influences her reproductive physiology. In 1979 Gershon Levinson and Sol Shnider at the University of California in San Francisco published findings that linked maternal fear to dysfunctional labor patterns. One year later, Roberto Sosa, M.D., and his associates published research in *The New England Journal of Medicine* suggesting that the presence of a person who offered emotional support to the mother decreased the length of labor and enhanced mother/infant bonding immediately after birth. This kind of research helped to humanize standard hospital procedures. Hospital birthing rooms that provided for labor and delivery in one place became increasingly available in the late 1970s and early 1980s. Women were permitted to have family members present during labor and to keep their babies with them after delivery. Family-centered birth became an option for women with low-risk pregnancies.

An unfriendly setting and insufficient emotional support can cause anxiety during labor, as can unrealistic childbirth preparation and negative feelings about impending motherhood. If a woman is at ease with her ability to mother, her family relationships, and the anticipated change in her lifestyle, she will be able to turn her attention to preparation for labor as childbirth approaches. Whether she readies herself for a natural birth or plans to use medication, she will need to develop skills for coping with pain. The more her expectation reflects the reality of birth, the less chance she will be shocked by an experience that is much harder and more intense than she had imagined.

Medical research has shown that fear can affect labor by decreasing blood levels of oxytocin, the hormone that causes contractions. I have found that a realistic, body-centered preparation helps a woman to integrate the intensity of labor even before it occurs. Body-centered preparation allows a woman to anticipate her own physical and emotional response to labor, to master her fear, and thus to give herself greater potential for a smooth and uncomplicated childbirth.

How a woman experiences childbirth may affect her confidence in the first days and weeks of mothering. Medical researchers John Kennell, Marshall Klaus, and M.A. Trause have shown that the hours and days immediately after birth are a sensitive period for mother/infant bonding. How the mother feels about her birth experience, no matter what course labor takes, may affect her relationship with her child. In my own clinical practice, I have observed that even years afterward women can reap psychological benefit from understanding their childbirth experience.

This book represents a continuation of my efforts to make childbirth an empowering and positive experience for women everywhere. Giving birth is the beginning of a mother's relationship with her child. It is also an opportunity for her personal growth.

What You Will Learn   Over the last seventeen years I have developed a method of childbirth preparation. It is a synthesis of my practical experience working with birthing mothers and their families and clinical research on how emotions affect labor. Giving birth is an experience carried not only into the first days of motherhood but also throughout life, having far-reaching effects on the mother's self-esteem and confidence.

This workbook, based on the method I use in my own

practice, augments physical and psychological preparations for labor; helps you explore your personal history, feelings, and anxieties about childbirth; and equips you with skills that maximize your potential for normal delivery. It should be used in the order it is written, skipping those exercises that do not pertain to your situation. In this workbook you will learn how to confront your fears, heal your past, and prepare for the best labor possible. You will learn how to do the following:

• Resolve emotional concerns about giving birth and becoming a mother. You will be able to identify childhood feelings about your parents that will help you to understand your own experience of giving birth and becoming a mother. The birth inventory in chapter 1 and the exercises in chapter 2 will help you confront fears, identify feelings, and achieve the self-knowledge so important to a calm and confident approach to labor.

• Overcome fear caused by your own birth or your previous childbirths. Through the visualization exercises and journal writing described in chapters 3 and 4 you can begin to heal prior birth and childbirth experiences that adversely affect your attitude and expectations for the upcoming delivery. Chapter 4 will also help you counteract cultural influences that negatively affect your feelings about childbirth.

• Prepare realistically for labor. The exercises in chapter 5 will prepare you for handling the different stages of labor. You will learn to let your body lead you into labor and to keep your mind from getting in the way with nonproductive anticipation. You will also learn how to develop attitudes and beliefs conducive to normal delivery. Exercises for increasing a couple's communication to help deal with labor and a guide for including siblings at birth are found in chapter 6. Chapter 7 explains how to identify your individual coping style and presents new techniques for coping with the pain of labor.

• Develop confidence in your ability to give birth and to mother your child. In chapter 8 you will be guided through a relaxation-and-birth visualization that addresses your unique concerns and situation. You will be given suggestions for creating personalized imagery and messages that will strengthen your resources for handling labor. Birth visualization will also help you bond with your baby before he or she is born.

• Maximize bonding with your baby immediately after birth and establish patterns for healthy family bonding. Chapter 9 gives suggestions for bonding with your new baby after delivery. Chapter 10 offers exercises for nurturing yourself and your relationship with your partner and establishing healthy family patterns for the year following the birth of your child.

What You Will Need Many of the exercises in this workbook are meant to be shared with your partner or another supportive person. Sometimes you will merely want to express your feelings. At other times you may find it useful or necessary to ask someone to assist you. Include your partner as often as possible and adjust the exercises to your current family and support network, including as many people as you wish. Participation will help your partner grow into his role as father. (I have used the term *partner* rather than *husband* in order to cover all possible family constellations.)

You will need a pen or pencil, a tape recorder for recording visualization sequences if you wish, and two blank sixty-minute audiocassettes to be used for the birth visualization in chapter 8 and other exercises. Comfortable clothing in which you can relax and lie down is also recommended.

The best place to use the workbook is one in which you feel safe and free of inhibitions. An optimal setting feels nurturing to you in some way, is relatively quiet, and is conducive to relaxation and closing your eyes. You should arrange not to be interrupted during the exercises. Your environment should provide you with enough privacy that you and your partner can talk about personal and intimate feelings as they arise.

The information and guided exercises in this workbook enhance your basic prenatal care by addressing your personal fears and anxieties. Doing these guided exercises is likely to help you experience a smooth labor. If medical intervention is needed during labor, however, you will be better prepared to cope with and adapt to the situation at hand. The ability to manage anxiety in a stressful situation can contribute greatly to your own health and the health of your baby.

In working through this book, you provide yourself an opportunity to strengthen your internal resources. The birth of your baby is the birth of your own motherhood. The baby now inside your womb will soon be cradled in your arms.

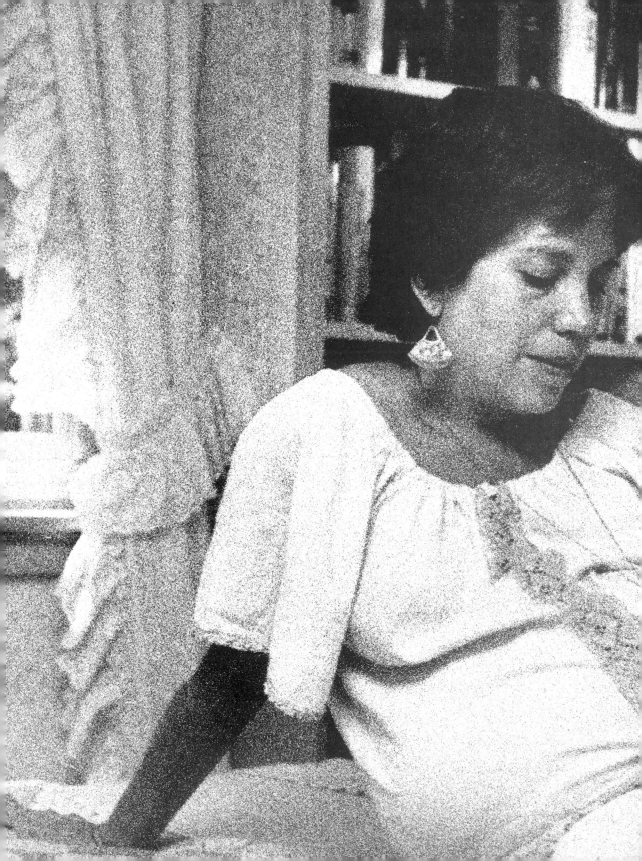

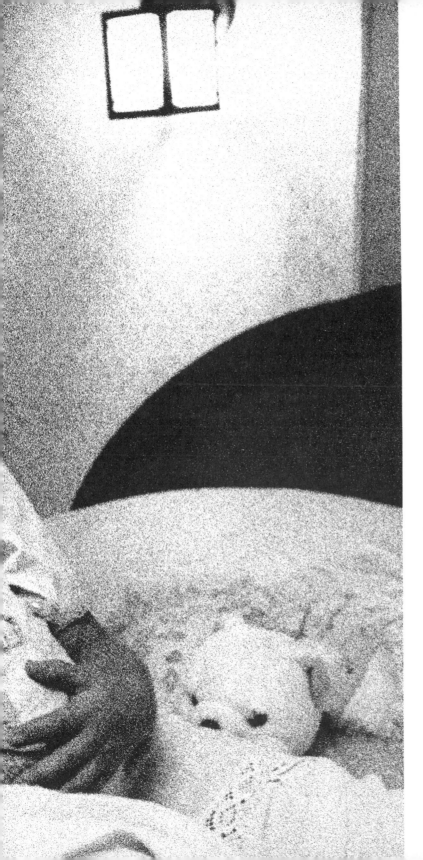

1

Your Birth Inventory

*If you have many painful feelings
to work through, you may fear that
doing so in pregnancy may harm
your baby. Since these feelings exist
inside you anyway, it will be an
advantage to release them and
clear the way for enjoyable
motherhood. . . . When you give
birth you will find it easier to let
go if you are not attempting to
control or suppress your
feelings. . . .*

JANET BALASKAS
Natural Pregnancy

PREGNANCY IS AN EMOTIONAL period. You are pregnant not only with new life, but also with feelings, expectations, and desires. Bringing forth new life is full of healthy stress. Stress can become distress, however, if you do not receive emotional support through this transition. Hormonal changes help ready you for motherhood by making you more emotionally sensitive. Your emotional vulnerability is your ally in bringing your feelings to the surface.

If you pay attention to the feelings generated during pregnancy and seek to understand and express your own needs throughout this transformative process, you will find yourself engaged in self-discovery. This is the emotional work of pregnancy. Your pregnancy provides you with new feelings and ideas about your future. It also brings up childhood memories. Exploring these feelings and memories readies you to greet your baby at birth. The emotional work of pregnancy nurtures the evolving new mother within you.

The birth-preparation inventory is a personal catalog of your feelings about the upcoming birth, designed to stimulate awareness of any anxiety you have about childbirth. You may begin by writing the answers to the questions here in the workbook, or you may prefer to use a journal set aside for this purpose. Sharing your written answers with your partner or a special friend can be helpful. (Later exercises require that you share your experience with someone you trust.) Some of the questions involve research, such as asking your mother for details about your own birth or contacting someone else who has this information.

You embark on an inward journey when you take time to reflect on your own birth, your previous childbirth experience, if any, and your hopes and expectations for this birth. Answering the questions in this chapter can increase self-awareness and deepen your resources for dealing with the life transition you are about to face. Such awareness will help you clarify your needs and maximize your benefit from the exercises in the rest of the workbook. Focusing on your emotional growth and change contributes to a smoother adjustment to labor and delivery.

Occasionally women feel emotional discomfort as they answer these questions. In the unusual case that your feelings are particularly disturbing or remain strong even after the exercise, you may want to seek professional counseling or psychotherapy. A supportive professional can be a valuable aid when needed, and pregnancy is a fertile time for personal growth. Whatever benefits you at this time will directly affect the generations that follow you, just as prior generations have affected your own growth and development.

1. Was this a planned pregnancy? _____

_____

_____

Birth-Preparation Inventory

2. What was your initial response when you realized you were pregnant? Have there been any changes in your attitude or feelings since then? _____

_____

_____

_____

_____

3. How has this pregnancy affected your relationships with your partner and other family members? _____

_____

_____

_____

_____

4. How will a baby fit into your current lifestyle and plans?

_____

_____

_____

5. Will a baby alter your lifestyle significantly or change your long-term plans? If so, how? _____

_____

_____

_____

6. What are your impressions and expectations of a newborn?

_____

_____

_____

_____

7. How will you and your partner share responsibility for the baby during the first year? _____

_____

_____

_____

_____

8. What do you know about your own birth? What is your impression of your mother's experience of childbirth? _____

_____

_____

_____

9. If you have given birth previously, what was it like for you? Is there anything you would change if you could? Is there anything you would do similarly the next time you give birth? _____

_____

_____

_____

_____

_____

10. Do you feel satisfied with your current plans for this childbirth? _____

_____

_____

11. How do you envision the birth of this baby? What is important to you? Who will be present at the birth? _____

_____

_____

_____

12. *How do you think you will cope with pain during labor? How do you want to prepare for labor?* _____

_____

_____

_____

13. *Do you like your body? Do you trust your body's changes during pregnancy and childbirth?* _____

_____

_____

_____

_____

14. *Do you have any particular concerns about this baby? About childbirth? About the postpartum period?* _____

_____

_____

_____

_____

Support and Sharing

Now that you have had time to think about these aspects of your life, choose someone with whom you can review the questionnaire, sharing your answers and discussing any feelings that arose. Pick someone whom you know will offer warmth and understanding—not judgment, critcism, or advice.

Ask the person to read the questions to you, then respond by saying your answers aloud. The other person should simply listen to you and repeat what is necessary to ensure that you are clearly understood.

This is an important part of the exercise as it encourages you to depend on someone else for support and sharing. The ability to share feelings can be a great asset during labor, so begin now to develop a relationship with a support person. Emotional support is not a luxury but, rather, an important part of your care during pregnancy, birth, and the postpartum period.

Emotional support can also improve the outcome of both labor and delivery. Research by Robert Sosa, M.D., and his associates at Childrens' Hospital in Cleveland, Ohio, found that the presence of a supportive companion shortened labor and increased the mother's ability to respond to her newborn immediately after birth. They write: "These observations suggest that there may be major perinatal benefits of constant human support during labor." But why wait until labor to begin this very beneficial process? In my experience, emotional support and sharing during pregnancy prepares a woman to cope with labor. She is less likely to be surprised by feelings that come up during labor when she has explored them during pregnancy.

Researchers Ellen Hodnett, Ph.D., R.N., and Richard Osborne, Ph.D., cite emotional support as the major factor in decreasing a woman's need for medication during labor. You will find it easier to cope if you can transform your feelings into words with the encouragement of an empathic listener. Writing in your journal also provides a way to become more aware of your feelings.

Feelings about past and present family relationships arise as you plan your own family. The following questionnaire assesses your emotional preparation for labor. Give yourself time to reflect on family relationships, your own readiness for motherhood, feelings about any previous childbirth, your experience of your mother's childbirths, your relationship to your body, the timing of this child, your current relationship with your partner, your satisfaction with your prenatal caregivers, your satisfaction with your present birth plans, and the quality of your support network.

Preparing for Labor   Rate the following on a scale from 0 to 5 (0 being very negative and 5 being very positive).

A. *Your relationship with your mother*

0   1   2   3   4   5   *current*

0   1   2   3   4   5   *childhood experience*

0. very painful, little or no contact, absence or abandonment as the major association

1. negative feelings predominate

2. nurturing in some ways, but with frequent struggle or misunderstanding

3. *positive feelings, but ambivalent about spending too much time with her*
4. *mostly positive feelings of warmth and understanding, with minor disagreement and little difficulty in communicating*
5. *very positive warm feelings, with a sense of closeness and respect for each other's differences*

B. *Your relationship with your father*
  current   0   1   2   3   4   5
  childhood experience   0   1   2   3   4   5

0. *very painful, little or no contact, absence or abandonment as the major association*
1. *negative feelings predominate*
2. *nurturing in some ways, but with frequent of struggle or misunderstanding*
3. *positive feelings, but ambivalent about spending too much time with him*
4. *mostly positive feelings of warmth and understanding, with minor disagreement and little difficulty in communicating*
5. *very positive warm feelings, with a sense of closeness and respect for each other's differences*

C. *Your childhood experience with siblings*   0   1   2   3   4   5

0. *antagonistic*
1. *emotionally distant*
2. *ambivalent but nurturing*
3. *satisfactory and nurturing*
4. *very rewarding despite minor dissatisfaction*
5. *highly satisfying, emotionally close and respectful*

D. *Your feelings of readiness for motherhood*   0   1   2   3   4   5

0. *completely unready, a mistake*
1. *mostly unready*
2. *ready, but with fear of inadequacy*
3. *mostly ready*
4. *ready and looking forward to it*
5. *ready and wishing it were already here*

0 1 2 3 4 5   **E.** *Your feelings about previous childbirth experiences or, if none, your understanding of your mother's experiences*

0. *very negative, frightening*
1. *negative, disappointing, emotionally traumatic*
2. *slightly negative but tolerable*
3. *hard but felt supported through it*
4. *difficult but enjoyable in retrospect*
5. *highly rewarding and positive event*

0 1 2 3 4 5   **F.** *Your relationship with your body, confidence about giving birth*

0. *lack of trust due to history of body ailments and sickness, fear of body processes*
1. *weakness, lack of confidence, dislike*
2. *slightly negative feelings*
3. *positive feelings, but some fear of weakness*
4. *strong and confident, mostly positive feelings*
5. *loving, nurturing, strong*

0 1 2 3 4 5   **G.** *Your feelings about having a baby at this time*

0. *terrible timing, will delay many personal plans*
1. *untimely, some delay of personal goals*
2. *untimely, but will work out*
3. *timely, but will be difficult to fit into lifestyle*
4. *good timing, will fit into plans well but take some reorganization*
5. *perfect timing, fits right in*

0 1 2 3 4 5   **H.** *Your feelings about integrating motherhood into your life, including your career*

0. *extremely difficult*
1. *very difficult*
2. *difficult, but expect it to get easier as child grows*
3. *fairly smooth*
4. *realistic and easy*
5. *easy and looking forward to the change*

I. *Your relationship with your partner*   0   1   2   3   4   5

0. antagonistic
1. negative and distant
2. slightly negative, but many positive attributes
3. satisfying
4. very satisfying, warm and close
5. highly satisfying, fulfilling

J. *Your current support network*   0   1   2   3   4   5

0. very isolated and alone
1. isolated, but making some connections
2. some relationships, somewhat supportive
3. supportive relationships
4. satisfying, supportive relationships
5. highly fulfilling and supportive relationships

K. *Your current birthing plans, including relationships with your*
    prenatal care givers   0   1   2   3   4   5

0. unsatisfactory, feel unsafe or antagonistic
1. unsatisfactory, feel safe but disrespectful
2. satisfactory plans, but little connection to care givers
3. satisfactory relationships, but plans still need to be worked out
4. satisfactory, with positive feelings for care givers and agreement
    about plans
5. satisfactory, with positive anticipation and nurturing relation-
    ship with care givers

Any feelings of dissatisfaction related to these topics
need your attention now. In the space provided or in your
journal, write the feelings you rated as minimally satisfactory or dissatisfying. Only by bringing these concerns to
the forefront of your attention can you begin to change
the beliefs, expectations, and plans that are unsatisfactory
to you.

_____

_____

_____

_____

_____

_____

_____

_____

Remember, it is not too late to make changes in your birth plans. Talking with your partner, arranging for marital counseling, expressing your needs to your care givers—all are ways of changing your life to make your pregnancy and delivery a more satisfying experience. Let your own needs and feelings be your guide. Write down any ideas you have for bringing more satisfaction, healing, or contentment to these areas of your life.

_____

_____

_____

_____

_____

_____

_____

_____

Now you can begin to take an inventory of factors that are important to you during this life transition. List the concerns that you wish to address as you work through the exercises in this book. You may want to change the list as you get closer to labor, so date your entry and plan to update it when you get to the exercise on birth visualization in chapter 8. By that time you will be more clear about what factors will increase your confidence for labor and motherhood. Briefly describe any anxiety you may have about the following:

1. Previous childbirth or your mother's childbirth history ____

_____

_____

2. Your own birth _____
_____
_____

3. Your age; career _____
_____
_____
_____
_____

4. Loss or abandonment in childhood; adulthood. These issues may include parental divorce, death, negatively charged relationship with a parent, or concerns about early childhood relationships and their effect on your parenting of your own child _____
_____
_____
_____
_____
_____

5. Being out of control during labor; pain during labor ____
_____
_____
_____
_____
_____

6. Anything else (present family relationships, spouse, sibling adjustment, etcetera) _____
_____
_____
_____
_____

Now list any associations that will support you during labor, including all the ratings of 5 that you circled in "Preparing for Labor." Note, for example, if a previous childbirth was rewarding and joyful, if your mother's story of your birth gives you feelings of warmth and happiness, if your parental relationships were supportive and nurturing, if you are already looking forward to the experience of labor, if you are surrounded by a supportive community, if you enjoy a deep and satisfying relationship with your partner, if you can already visualize your family bonding with love and excitement, if you are feeling empowered by pregnancy, if you are enjoying your sensuality and bodily changes. . . . Include all positive feelings that were highlighted or brought to your awareness as you answered the questionnaire.

_____

_____

_____

_____

_____

_____

_____

_____

_____

_____

_____

As you work through this book pay special attention to issues that move you intensely. Those that are not of particular concern, you may ignore. Participate only in the exercises that apply to your current needs. For example, if you never experienced a difficult childbirth, skip the exercise in chapter 4 on healing previous childbirth trauma. You may also find it useful to refer to the case study of Terri in appendix 1 to help you create your own birth inventory.

As you worked through this chapter you became aware of the feelings you carry with you on your present journey to motherhood. Keep in mind that expressing your feelings releases tension. Feelings are physical. Research shows that women who habitually store uncomfortable feelings rather than expressing them experience more difficult labors. Talking with your partner or a friend and writing in a journal helps you move through the changes of pregnancy.

Not only will your body tension lessen, but you will have taken the first step toward resolving emotional conflicts. Acknowledging feelings is one way humans adapt to change.

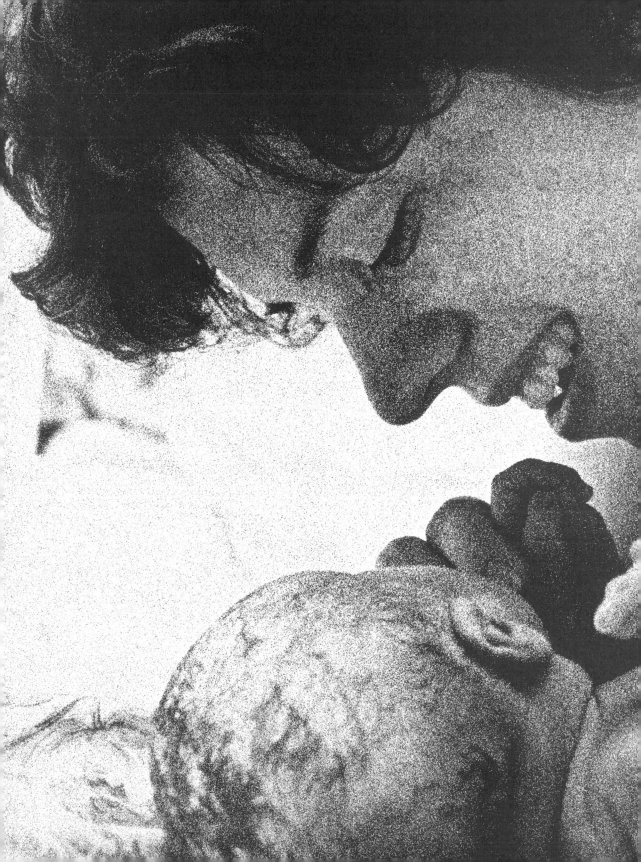

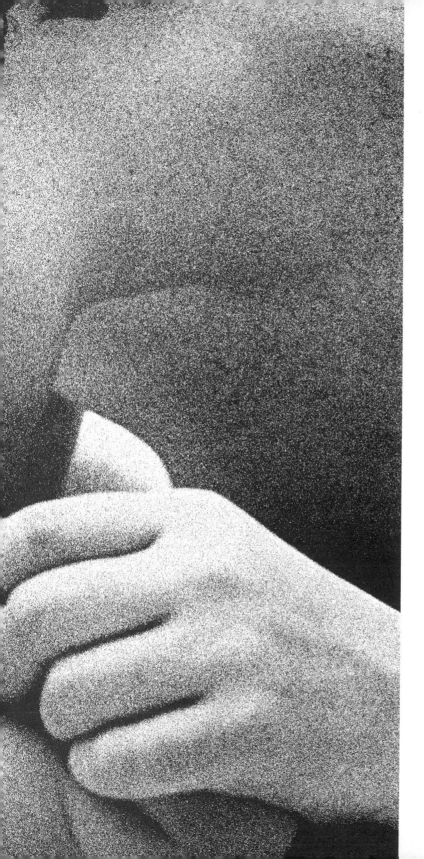

2

Becoming
a Mother

*I secretly feared the trials and
tribulations of parenthood when I
was pregnant with my first
child . . . yet now that I have
become a mother it is almost
impossible to describe the pleasure
and depth it can bring to
living. . . .*

RENÉE
mother of four

BECOMING A MOTHER IS a life transition that our culture greatly underestimates. Few other life changes are as complete and irreversible, and few life events provoke as much ambivalence. I know of no other experience that simultaneously stimulates two powerfully divergent fantasies: the promise of ultimate fulfillment and the threat of selfless sacrifice. Somewhere in between lies the reality of motherhood.

Pregnancy is a journey. At the end, a woman gives birth not only to a baby, but also to her own identity as a mother. Pregnancy is, therefore, an emotional and psychological as well as a physiological transformation.

Your adjustment to pregnancy and labor is enhanced when you express your anxieties about the demands of motherhood. If your concerns remain buried or denied, or if your fears about childbirth are ignored or minimized, the inevitable natural stresses of labor and delivery may intensify these anxieties.

Gershon Levinson and Sol Shnider at the University of California at San Francisco School of Medicine found that anxiety during labor limited the release of oxytocin, a hormone that stimulates contractions, resulting in dysfunctional laboring patterns. Fear in labor may also contribute to a reduction in the supply of oxygen to the baby. Many scientific studies have documented the impact of emotional variables on the labor process, yet medicine has almost never offered women a means for coping with these natural anxieties, perhaps assuming that fear was abnormal and therefore beyond normal prenatal care. In fact, anxiety during the transitional period is common, but women are seldom given an opportunity to discuss the meaning of this transition. Prenatal care providers rarely recognize that the physical process of childbirth is intertwined with a woman's concern not only about labor, but also about the changes that having a baby will bring to life beyond the delivery room.

When you explore your feelings about motherhood, you can overcome anxieties about childbirth. Expressing your feelings through writing and through exercises shared with your partner can help you release the tension caused by unspoken fears.

Remember that pregnancy is a period of psychological, physical, and emotional upheaval. This means that you may have feelings of excitement and trepidation about motherhood, expectations for fulfillment, and fear of future deprivation. All these feelings are natural. It is necessary for some women to mourn the loss of a lifestyle in which they felt free and spontaneous, without responsibilities for a child. But feelings are not actions. Because you feel this way at times does not mean you want to change your mind or send your baby back. This sense of loss is not a feeling you need to do anything about. Simply recognizing ambivalence as a normal part of decision making can banish any guilt you might otherwise create for yourself. Sadness about the past will be replaced by the excitement of anticipation if you can allow yourself to say goodbye to your old life. By acknowledging fear, loss, or disappointment, you make way for joy, love, and hope for the future.

Assuming responsibility for another human life also brings up feelings of vulnerability. During pregnancy it is natural to feel more dependent, particularly on your partner. The desire to be taken care of arises as you adapt to your body's many changes. Feeling dependent on your mate or other people may then bring up fears of abandonment. Working through this fear, perhaps talking with your partner about these feelings, will pave the way for adjustment to the family unit you are creating. If you communicate your fears, you minimize the likelihood of drifting apart. In the years ahead you will need to depend on one another in your new roles as parents.

Loss and Vulnerability: Normal Feelings

Some women feel increasingly sensual during their pregnancy while others, feeling unattractive, lose their interest in sex. Hormone changes may increase your sexual drive, yet you may feel vulnerable to rejection from your partner and need reassurance that you are still sexually appealing in your new pregnant shape. Remember you are not fat, but pregnant! A man may experience a range of confusing feelings as he adjusts to his wife becoming a mother. Combining sexual feelings for you as a lover with the feelings he may have about motherhood can be a difficult adjustment.

Sex and Sensuality During Pregnancy

Still, pregnancy can be a time of increased sexual intimacy. Sexual activity cannot hurt your baby as long as the pregnancy is following a normal course. In fact, sexuality is a healthy part of pregnancy. Get to know your new shape. Aquaint yourself with your pregnant body through activities you find sensual and enjoyable. Sharing warm baths, taking turns massaging oil on your growing abdomen, and enjoying a healthy sexual relationship can bring you and your partner closer at this time. Your pregnancy is a temporary state. Allow yourself to enjoy it.

Mother/Daughter Relationship

Besides physical changes causing feelings of dependency, the journey toward parenthood stirs up deep desires to be mothered yourself. Your relationship with your own mother comes up for review as you develop your own identity as a mother. The kind of relationship you had with her may have influenced whatever confidence you have in your own abilities to mother. This new being will depend on you for its very life; now you will be the powerful influence. Your child's life and much of his or her future development is in your hands. Some women feel confident and ready for this responsibility and others do not. It is natural for you to feel excited by the challenge of parenting, to anticipate the joys and rewards. It is also normal to feel anxiety about the job that awaits you.

Will I Be a Good Mother?

Fears of inadequacy often result from an overburdened childhood. If you were in a caretaking role with your own parents, you may have taken on more responsibility than you were capable of as a child. One client, Cynthia, was the first of eight children. She feared she would be inadequate as a parent. When we helped her explore her background it became clear to her that she had been given overwhelming responsibilities for her seven siblings. In her teens she had begged her mother not to have any more children because as the eldest she couldn't handle the workload. I helped Cynthia see that her age at that time was inappropriate for mothering. Now, however, she really was an adult, and her responsibilities would be proportionate to her level of maturity. I compared her being a twelve-year-old carrying around a 125-pound baby (her mother) to her being a thirty-six-year-old carrying a normal seven-pound child. The comparison helped her understand that she could separate her previous negative mothering experience from what was possible for her now. She was able to grieve the loss of her childhood freedom. Expressing the sadness enabled her to understand her postponement of childbearing until later in life. She had wanted those years of freedom to take care of her own needs. After considering all this, she began to feel confident about her own capacity to mother.

Fears of inadequacy in mothering may also stem from a negative relationship with your own mother. Working through your feelings about this relationship will reward you with an understanding of what you want to carry into your own mothering and what you do not. Like everyone else, you were influenced by your upbringing, but the awareness of these feelings frees you to create your own parent/child relationships differently. Although you will, no doubt, have many positive and nurturing feelings that you wish to carry forward from the past, you will develop your own style based on your own needs and personality. No two mothers are identical, and no parent/child relationship is entirely predictable.

You depend on your childhood relationship with your mother as a guide for developing your own style of mothering. This doesn't mean that you necessarily copy your mother's style or that you want to replicate your relationship with her. The psychological task of becoming a mother is to sort through your past, keeping what you want and letting go of what you do not wish to pass on to the next generation.

You may feel particularly vulnerable if you never received the nurturing you needed as a child. Feelings of love as well as anger may emerge as you do the following exercise, which will help you to acknowledge feelings about your relationship with your parents. It may also stimulate discussion between you and your partner about the parents you want to be. Don't forget that your relationship with your father was also important. You will draw from your relationships with both parents when you envision the kind of mother you want to be. You may be aware of other role models in your past. Aunts, uncles, babysitters, grandmothers, and grandfathers may have contributed to your resources for mothering.

Becoming a Parent   Ask your partner or a friend to read the questions listed here, inserting your name in the blanks and interviewing you as if you were your mother. Answer the questions spontaneously. Trust that whatever you say holds some emotional meaning for you, even if it is not necessarily the truth about your relationship. Later, you may want to ask your mother these questions and compare your own answers to those she gives. The value of this exercise lies in your own interpretations of your childhood. Whatever comes up will be what you feel now, as you are becoming a mother. Your answers will speak the truth about your own feelings of being mothered. Ask your partner to listen to your answers supportively and attentively, to comfort you if necessary, and to laugh with you as well.

1. What was your experience of giving birth to _____ _____ *?*

2. What kind of a baby was your daughter, _____ *?*

3. What was it like to raise _____ *?*

4. What was most difficult for you in raising _____ _____ *?*

5. What was easy about raising _____ *?*

6. If you could do it over again, is there anything you would do differently in raising _____ *?*

7. How do you feel about _____ *having a baby now?*

8. Do you think _____ *will be a good parent?*

Our interpretation of how our parents raised us forms the blueprint for our own expectations and beliefs about parenting. You may feel very loved by your mother and confident of your own ability to parent. Or you may feel that your mother was lacking in some way—something you want to provide for your own child. Awareness of the source of your strong feelings will allow you greater freedom to form healthy relationships with your children. An overwhelming desire to make up for your own early pain may nonetheless cause you to wound your child. For example, if your mother's style of discipline was overly strict, and you have unresolved feelings of hurt and anger, you may feel deeply committed to permissiveness. Since your own child cannot feel the pain you endured during childhood, however, he or she may experience your leniency as lack of discipline or even neglect. Once you are aware of your own wounds, you can heal them without projecting your unmet needs onto your child.

Whatever attitudes toward parenting your mother expressed will be a part of your heritage. What decisions will you make about the kind of mother you want to be? Are there things you would do the same? Differently?

Repeat the previous exercise, starting with the second question, as you stand in for your father. Then take time to share your feelings about him. What did you like about your relationship with him? What did you dislike? Is there anything about his fathering you would want to change for your own child? Or do the same? Repeat the full exercise with your partner, asking him questions about himself as if he were his father. Then repeat the questions, having him role-play his mother. Listen sensitively and supportively to his answers. Comfort him if necessary and be ready to laugh with him as well.

Adapt this exercise to your particular circumstances. You can repeat it with a supportive friend and compare your family experiences. Find out what you can learn from your friends. If you are a single parent, identify someone you can depend on for emotional support in parenting. Many single mothers can benefit from friends who want involvement with a child without taking full responsibility for one of their own.

Discuss together the blueprints for parenting that you and your partner received. You can use the following questions as a guide for discussion.

What were the messages you received about yourself from each of your parents? Were they accurate or not? How did you feel about these messages?

What strengths do you bring to parenting from your childhood experiences?

What weaknesses do you bring to parenting from your childhood experiences?

How will you and your partner help each other with parenting?

How do you see yourselves working as a parenting team to nurture each other and your child?

How do you feel about each other as parents?

What are your feelings about raising a boy? about raising a girl?

What kind of mother or father do you think your partner will be?

What feelings did this exercise bring up for you?

Each of you will bring strengths to parenting and each of you will bring weaknesses. Find out what these are and plan to help each other with your respective blind spots. For example, if you feel you may be overly critical, or you see that your partner overcompensates for his father's strictness by never saying no, discuss these concerns now. Your communication can strengthen your relationship and bring you a sense of security and confidence that will benefit you during labor.

Mothering Yourself Finding your own way as a mother means that you must take your needs as well as your baby's into account. Lyn DelliQuadri, M.S.W., and Kati Breckenridge, Ph.D., in their book *The New Mother Care* recommend that women develop an attitude of self-care in the early stages of mothering. It is difficult, if not impossible, to attend to the needs of your child if you do not take care of your own. Good mothering is not perfect mothering. Achieving a balance of the needs of all family members is the key to good-enough mothering, a concept developed by D.W. Winnicott—a British psychoanalyst and pediatrician who studied the influence of mothering on child development. DelliQuadri and Breckenridge sum up Winnicott's philosophy:

The concept [of good-enough mothering] is a practical replacement for the idealized standards of the mother myths and the contradictory theories of the experimental psychologists, because it tells us that the activities of mothering can be performed in many different ways and still provide basic, "good enough" care.

Both the nurturing and the wounds you received as a child have prepared you for the challenges of raising your child in your own way. During pregnancy and after, you will be discovering and defining your own approach to mothering. There is no magic formula. The most you can achieve is a balance between your needs and the needs of your child and other family members. Rest assured that your child does not expect you to be perfect. Your child shares in your growth and fulfillment. As you consider what is best for your child, keep yourself in mind. Your child will benefit from your happiness in life.

Mothers Have Needs, Too

Many pregnant women fear they will lose themselves in motherhood. Although it is true that the demands on you will be great, you can look forward to developing your own interests, and you can pursue goals you have set for yourself. Motherhood can strengthen your ability to cope and provide you with a new appreciation of life. Your needs as a person are important to the health and development of the family. You must take your needs seriously. Integrating your needs with your baby's and finding a balance that works is fundamental to family happiness. The following exercise will help you set priorities as you enter motherhood.

Write down five activities, pursuits, or interests that are important for you to maintain in the year following childbirth. Promise yourself that you will look at this list again in the month after your baby is born. This way you can remind yourself of the personal interests you want to integrate with motherhood.

_____

_____

_____

_____

_____
_____
_____
_____
_____
_____
_____
_____
_____
_____
_____
_____
_____
_____
_____
_____
_____
_____
_____
_____

Becoming a mother does not need to rob you of your selfhood. Stay away from martyrdom. Martyrs never make good mothers; what is gained in giving is taken away in guilt.

The Changing Family The birth of a baby cannot be viewed as an isolated event; it is a family event. Whether a baby is greeted with love, joy, fear, or trepidation depends both on circumstances immediately surrounding the birth and on much that has come before.

Social scientists say the American family is in a state of crisis. Changing cultural roles for women and the challenges of blended and single-parent families add to the adjustments already needed when new life is brought forth. Financial and caretaking responsibilities are now shared more equally between the sexes. This change has given women new freedom, but it has also produced conflicts for those pulled between the demands of family and career.

None of these situations may affect you personally, but changes in society at large influence the way you experience motherhood. When the very definition of family is fluid, it is natural that women feel insecure. Today many women delay motherhood until their careers and relationships are firmly in place. The postponement creates another set of challenges: Established lifestyles must shift as women sort through their need to work and their desire to stay home with their infants. Is it any wonder that women giving birth today need special support?

First-time Mothers Over Thirty-Five

Since 1982 there has been a dramatic increase in the number of women having first babies at age thirty-five and later. Baby boomers, those born between 1946 and 1964 are entering their later childbearing years, and many of them have delayed motherhood. According to John Hansen, M.D., who reviewed the literature on maternal age and pregnancy outcome, these two factors were expected to increase the over–thirty-five age group's proportion of total births by 72 percent between 1982 and the turn of the century.

Statistics on pregnancy and labor outcome for first-time mothers older than thirty-five are varied and inconclusive. These women have a higher rate of complication during labor, including a greater number of Cesarean sections, but the research does not differentiate those who were healthy during pregnancy from those with medical problems, such as diabetes and toxemia. Most authorities agree that if you are generally healthy, exercise regularly, and maintain a healthy diet, your chances of having a normal labor should not be any different at thirty-five than at twenty-five. Statistics, however, do not address the special emotional concerns and stresses that affect the older woman.

These women bring a different perspective to parenthood. By the time they reach their mid-thirties, work and career have usually been paramount in their lives. Even when career goals are not a major concern, middle age is a very different time in the life cycle to give birth. Older women may feel greater loss of their unfettered lifestyle than do younger women. Financial arrangements in the marriage may shift dramatically if a woman who previously held a high-paying position is now staying home with her new baby. These changes may affect a woman's self-esteem and make for a more difficult adjustment to motherhood.

Finally, women having first babies later in life often waited because they had fearful expectations of motherhood. This was true for Cynthia, the woman who had cared for her seven younger siblings. Because of her own lost childhood, she was not ready to become a mother until she was thirty-six. Her reasons for waiting included unexpressed fears that she needed to understand before she became a mother. This is a different perspective from a twenty-four-year-old who enjoyed the freedom of childhood and is now ready to take on the adult responsibilities of parenthood. Not all women who wait until later in life to give birth are fearful, however it is possible that those who delay are in general more ambivalent. The threats of Down's syndrome and other genetic defects that increase with maternal age also contribute to their anxiety. Medical researchers have long overlooked the influence of life-change factors on the outcome of labor. In the quest to understand the higher complication rates for women over thirty-five, researchers have ignored the emotional lives of the women they study.

If you have concerns about finances, loss of your previous lifestyle, or the blending of family and career, you are among a fast-growing group of women. Your concerns are real and need to be addressed. Joining a support group and making daily entries in your journal will help you work through your fears. Sharing your anxieties with your partner and other women who are experiencing similar mid-life changes can make the difference between postpartum depression and a healthy adjustment to motherhood. Find out what resources are available in your community. Plan now to join a support group for mothers after your baby is born.

Freedom and Commitment in Motherhood

Ambivalence is a natural part of commitment. Working through your mixed feelings about becoming a mother is an important part of your journey. A friend once said to me that freedom and commitment are differentiated only by a verb; freedom is choice and commitment is to make a choice. You have made the choice to mother. Making choices is an inevitable part of growing up. Freedom becomes meaningless without commitment, and the choice to mother can be a profoundly rewarding commitment. Honor your feelings and remember that your ability to make such an important life decision means you can create meaning in your life. Write down your personal reasons for choosing motherhood. Take time to consider your feelings and thoughts about this decision.

_____

_____

_____

_____

_____

_____

_____

_____

_____

_____

_____

_____

_____

_____

_____

_____

_____

_____

_____

_____

_____

_____

_____

_____

_____

_____

Some of these reasons will be easy for you to write down, while other thoughts and feelings may be difficult to express in words. You may wish to come back to this list after you have experienced motherhood. Your decision to have a child will become increasingly meaningful to you in the years ahead, as you learn and grow with your baby, your child, and eventually your adolescent.

It is true that you often hear parents bemoan the trials of parenthood; however, it is almost impossible to express the pleasure and gratification that having a child can bring. To me, the following experience represents one of those nearly indescribable feelings. I was swinging gently in a hammock in my backyard, my seven-month-old son snuggled sleepily to my chest as we swayed rythmically side to side, listening to the birds, smelling the moist earth after a morning rain, when suddenly our rocking movement flipped us into the air. I arched my body instantly, maneuvering myself to land below my son rather than on top of him as gravity would have had it. He landed safely upon me. It was complete and instinctual love that enabled me to protect him with my body. In the mother/child relationship I discovered a capacity to love and defend that I had not known before. It is satisfying to care this deeply, but it is a difficult feeling to verbalize and share with others. Perhaps this is why it is more common to hear complaints about parenthood than expressions of the satisfaction that it can bring. In the days and weeks ahead, ask other parents what in their relationship with their children brings them pleasure and satisfaction.

If you are in your mid-thirties or older when you have your first baby, you bring the benefit of maturity to motherhood. Knowledge of yourself and others increases with age. Greater life experience allows you to appreciate the choice you have made to mother. You may have much more to give because you have waited. Love and bonding will deepen your commitment. Experience will be your teacher. Thinking about your reasons for becoming a mother may help you feel deeper, or renewed, certainty about your decision.

In the next two chapters you will explore the three major ways that you learned about childbirth and the effect this has on your own preparation for giving birth.

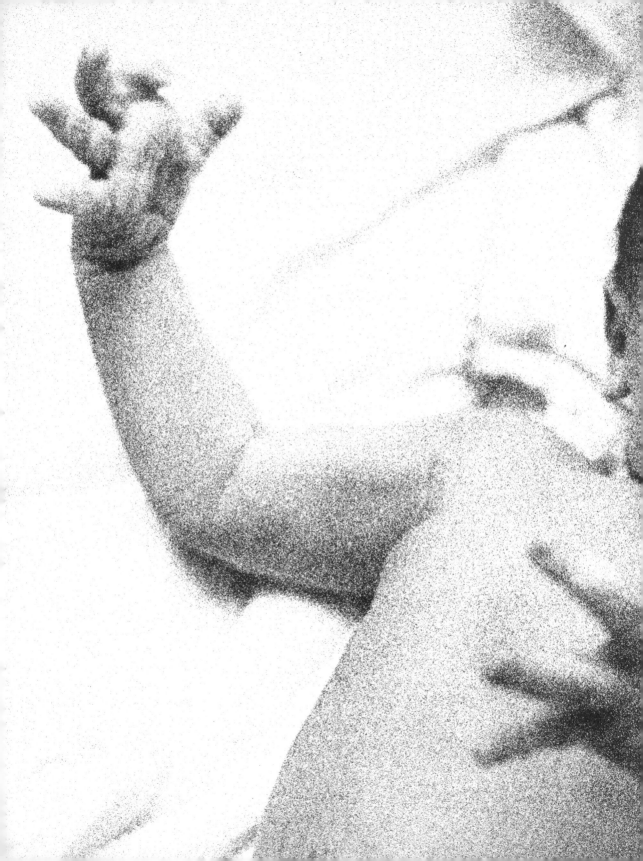

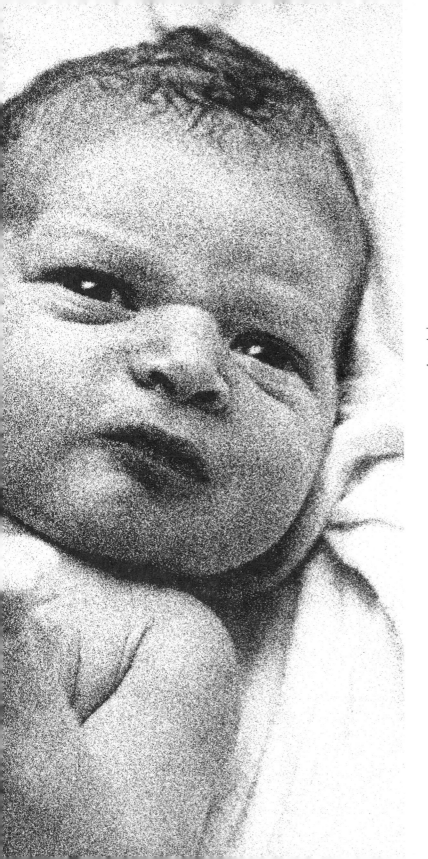

3

Being Born: Our First Experience of Birth

I came down the tunnel.
It was light. It was cold. . . .
ANNE
memory of her own birth

OUR INITIAL LEARNING TAKES place before we have words for it. Being born is our first experience of labor. We carry the memory in our bodies, and this body memory can affect our own childbearing. A painful or difficult entrance into the world can affect subliminal beliefs and expectations for labor and delivery.

A daughter's expectations of childbirth can also be affected by her mother's labor with her. Many pregnant women come to see me for help in resolving feelings about a difficult childbirth. These women often discover that the emotional themes present when they gave birth also appeared in their own birth history. Occasionally the experiences of mother and daughter seem contradictory, though the emotional impact is amazingly similar—as if the daughter is working through the difficulties experienced by her own mother at birth.

Lisa came to see me during her second pregnancy. She wanted help preparing for a vaginal delivery following a previous cesarean. Lisa had anticipated a home birth in her first pregnancy, but she developed high blood pressure as she neared her due date. She then hoped for a vaginal birth in the hospital but ended up with a cesarean because the doctor could not hear her baby's heartbeat. She feared for her baby's life, but when he emerged, her son was healthy. The doctor was not sure that the baby had suffered any difficulty at all. Another theme in Lisa's first childbirth was her great distress during the cesarean due to incomplete anesthesia. She was also shocked by the sudden upset of all her plans.

When I asked her about her own birth, we discovered some strikingly similar emotional themes. Her mother had been told that Lisa was not alive because the doctor could not find a heartbeat. Because of the rapidity of labor, Lisa's mother delivered naturally. Her mother had difficulty adjusting to labor. Although this was her third child, she had never experienced natural childbirth. She was left with an experience similar to Lisa's, but from the opposite perspective. She was upset by the turnaround from medicated delivery to natural birth. Like Lisa, her mother was surprised and relieved to discover that her baby was alive and well after all. At the end of our session together, Lisa reflected that it was as if she had experienced the cesarean that her mother had wanted during labor with her.

It is not uncommon to hear birth stories with similar themes generation after generation. By healing emotional pain generated during your own birth, you clear away unresolved emotions that may increase your anxieties during childbirth. Perhaps Lisa's unexpected rise in blood pressure at the end of an otherwise healthy pregnancy was precipitated by a preverbal memory of her own birth.

At birth we are too young to organize experience into cognitive memory. Nevertheless, our body remembers. Through hypnosis it is possible to get in touch with birth memory. Psychologist David Chamberlain and David Cheek, an obstetrician and hypnotist, believe that prenatal and birth memories can play an important role in our orientation toward the world. How we are born can have far-reaching effects on our attitudes and beliefs about ourselves. Sometimes our birth influences our perception of the world as a friendly place where people will meet our needs, sometimes as a hostile environment that must be controlled. In other cases, the experience of being born will only be reactivated during childbirth.

Birth Memory

We are concerned here with memories and associations that specifically affect your subliminal beliefs and expectations for childbirth. I use the term *subliminal* in the literal sense. It derives from the latin word *limen*, or threshold, and means *below the threshold of consciousness*. The memories we hold in our bodies, whether from our own birth or from previous childbirth, are not always congruent with what we learn intellectually in childbirth classes. We may tell ourselves that birth is a natural and safe process and recall our childbirth teacher's emphasis that a woman's body is designed for giving birth, but our own bodies may hold a different truth. It is essential to honor body memory, as it wields far more influence than the intellect during labor.

Preverbal birth memory can be stimulated physically and emotionally by childbirth; that is, labor and delivery will present an opportunity for your body memories to surface.

By processing such memories now you can understand and experience feelings separately from your upcoming childbirth. Becoming aware of any negative feelings about your own birth allows you to release tension that you otherwise might carry into labor.

In my clinical practice I often hear women referring to their own birth experience without being consciously aware that they are doing so. Vague fears, such as the feeling that descent through the birth canal will be fraught with danger, may surface only by tangential association. Judy, expecting her first baby, reported no concerns about childbirth and expressed the belief that birth was a safe and natural process, one she was looking forward to. As she reclined to do a birth visualization, however, she had great difficulty finding a comfortable position and jokingly said: "I'd better find the right position or the baby might suffocate on the way down." When I asked her what she knew about her own birth she said it had been her mother's second birth and that it had been a normal and relatively rapid labor. The next week she reported that her mother had called her on the telephone, so Judy had asked her more specifically about the delivery.

Judy learned that there had been much difficulty getting her out because her shoulders were stuck. When the doctor finally freed her, Judy had required resuscitation in order to breathe.

Judy had not been aware of any fears connected to her own birth, yet her body did not feel comfortable in any of the positions she assumed for the birth visualization and her offhand comment expressed the body memory she held beneath the threshold of conscious awareness. Her birth association surfaced only as she reclined to visualize the upcoming labor and birth. Such associations dance on the edges of our consciousness because they do not fit our intellectual preparation and because, as with Judy, there may be ignorance of the actual birth experience. The body, however, does not forget, and when associations close to that body memory are activated, they influence the way we approach our own labor and childbirth. If birth has been difficult or frightening, it is important to work through the fear until the pregnant woman can visualize travel through the birth canal as safe.

Healing may have already occurred through spontaneous child or adult play, such as crawling through tires, scuba diving through underwater caves and tunnels, or playing a game called coming down the vagina, as one mother did with her eighteen-month-old. Her son had been born by cesarean after showing signs of fetal distress. She assisted him in playing a game, repeatedly acting out a descent but this time through a turtle-neck sweater—the two of them laughing uncontrollably as he burrowed through the opening of the sweater into the bedcovers. Healing may take place in ways we are not aware of, but unresolved body memories inevitably will surface at the next childbirth. Perhaps this is the body's effort to heal psychic wounds. The greater the emotional charge, the more possibility there is that such memories will affect the present childbirth.

If your birth was a pleasant or joyful experience it carries a different impact. Positive memories of being born encourage the childbirth process. A woman with a body memory of sliding easily and safely through the vaginal doorway to loving, waiting arms has a subliminal association to birth as natural, healthy, and even exciting. This woman has a sense that everything will be fine. Her feeling goes beyond the intellect. Her perception of childbirth as a natural and do-able process is grounded in her own sensation of birth.

What Happened During My Birth?

It is no surprise that the demand for more natural and family-oriented birth arose among women whose mothers were so heavily medicated that they were "knocked out" for delivery. Most likely your mother received the routine care given to women before changes in obstetrical practice became widespread in the 1970s and 1980s. The standard practice was to separate the laboring woman from any support of family or friends, which often meant excluding the father-to-be as well. It was common for her to be left isolated to face one of her life's most intense and painful experiences. Drugs were administered to frightened and lonely women, as much to ease fear as to relieve pain.

Routine separation of mother and newborn followed, with fathers allowed to peer through nursery windows at their offspring. Families were not reunited until days after birth when, finally, the bonding could begin. If your mother did not have a natural childbirth, it is likely that you were born in such an atmosphere with some, if not all, of these customary procedures as a part of your birth experience. If so, you may have associations of abandonment at birth. You may have suffered the absence of loving arms to welcome you.

In his book *Babies Remember Birth*, David Chamberlain suggests that newborns do feel their mother's fears and that they experience despondency in prolonged separations from mother after birth. Women who were separated from their mothers may find, when it comes time to deliver their own babies, that they associate separation anxiety with childbirth.

Twenty years of medical research on alternative approaches to, childbirth, pressure from consumers, and increasing numbers of women delivering at home have forced changes in hospital policies. The medical community has responded to women's demands for access to family support, less drugs and fewer routine interventions, and opportunities for immediate family bonding. Birthing rooms have been set up within hospitals to provide a home-like setting for laboring mothers and their families.

There is still room for improvement in the obstetrical delivery system, but it is a far cry from the "twilight sleep" nightmare of our mothers or grandmothers' hospitalized deliveries and the customary separations that were at the heart of our mother's and our own beginnings. Now it is possible to give birth and have your baby with you immediately or soon after delivery. You can reassure yourself that an extended separation is not likely to be a part of your child's birth. Letting yourself feel your desire to welcome your baby at birth can help you heal your own anxiety about early separation.

If you were fortunate enough to have had a relatively natural birth, with little or no separation after delivery, consider yourself lucky. In the United States, you are one of a minority of your generation. If, however, you know your birth was routine, then you can assume there was some fear associated with your isolation in a hospital nursery and the absence of waiting arms. Naturally there will be a range of experience here from a very negative, hostile reception into the world to a warm and friendly welcome, depending on the hospital staff and your mother's or father's emotional and physical availability. Try to get a detailed and accurate description of your birth, including the emotional atmosphere surrounding your delivery and the several days or weeks until you arrived home.

The following questions can help you reconstruct the past and help you to get in touch with feelings about your own birth. Ask your mother or someone you think would know the answers to the following questions. Use these questions to prompt your own thinking and remembering. Begin to uncover the experience from your own perspective. What do you think birth was like for you? Write down what you know or what you believe to be the answers to the questions. Reconstruct the most accurate picture you can about the circumstances surrounding your own birth.

Remembering Your Birth

1. Were there any major transitions in the family during my mother's pregnancy with me? What were the living arrangements? Which family members were closely involved? What was my mother's emotional state? _____

_____

_____

_____

_____

_____

_____

_____

2. Was I planned? Wanted? _____

_____

_____

_____

_____

_____

_____

_____

3. *Was the pregnancy healthy?* _____

_____
_____
_____
_____
_____

4. *Was I a full-term baby? Premature? Overdue? Mother's emotional state immediately before delivery?* _____

_____
_____
_____
_____
_____
_____

5. *What was my delivery like? Complications? Length of labor?*

_____
_____
_____
_____
_____
_____

6. *What was Mother's state of consciousness at delivery?* __

_____
_____
_____
_____
_____
_____

7. *Was I healthy upon delivery? Complications after birth? Any unique circumstances, such as adoption?* _____

_____
_____
_____
_____
_____
_____

8. *Did anyone hold me after birth? What happened immediately afterward?* _____

_____

_____

_____

_____

_____

9. *When did my mother first see me? Hold me? Father? Other family members?* _____

_____

_____

_____

_____

_____

_____

10. *If I was in a nursery, what was the experience like? How long was I there following birth? Who fed me? How?* _____

_____

_____

_____

_____

_____

_____

11. *When did I come home?* _____

_____

_____

12. *What is Mother's first memory following birth? Father's?*

_____

_____

_____

_____

_____

_____

13. How does Mother describe my first year of life? Was it a happy time for her? Stressful, and if so how? Father's description?

_____

_____

_____

_____

_____

_____

After reflecting on the above questions and answers, write down five or more words that describe the way you as a baby may have experienced your birth and entrance into the world.

_____

_____

_____

After satisfying yourself that you have gathered the information available to you about your birth and your mother's labor, lean back and relax; take your time to connect with that baby that was you. What do you think that experience was like for you as a newborn? How might you have felt but lacked words to express? What did the family situation feel like to you, although you could not understand it as you can now? How might the physical sensations of labor and birth have felt to you then? What might it have felt like to be held? What might your mother have felt like to you? When did you feel comfortable and safe? Finally, close your eyes and imagine what your birth was like for you.

Your Birth Story Now write the best story you can about your own birth. Include things you know as well as things you sense as truth. Even if you could not obtain much information about your birth, write down your imagined sensations of the process. Trust that body memory will fill in what it can to help you.

_____

_____

_____

_____
_____
_____
_____
_____
_____
_____
_____
_____
_____
_____
_____
_____
_____
_____
_____
_____
_____
_____
_____
_____

You will probably have some very pleasant sensations and some that are unpleasant, depending on your personal history. Now go back to what you have written about the experience and imagine yourself inside your mother's womb, getting ready to be born, starting from the beginning again. Read the following exercise through before closing your eyes, leaning back, and relaxing into the suggestions.

A Positive Visualization of Your Own Birth

All the compassion that you have ever given anyone in your life, give to your little baby self, now. Assure the baby self that you are present and waiting for her. Your presence gives her a sense of safety and trust. Since this is your visualization exercise, you are in control of the outcome. Imagine what it could feel like to dive straight down the vagina—safe, warm, and stimulating! The rhythmic pressure of contractions and the movement through the birth canal help ready a baby for the outside world. If your baby self feels fear or danger, resolve these now in your visualization. Reassure and comfort her through any part of the journey that needs healing. As she makes her way down to the opening, tell her that the coolness *she feels on her head is the air outside and that she will adjust to it quickly as she slides through. And tell her that you are waiting to hold her in your arms, to love her and nurture her as she grows. Imagine what it feels like to be massaged down through the vagina, to have your head emerging, to turn your shoulders just right as you come into the world, sliding through, what it feels like to slide easily through the soft warmth into the world. Now play the part of your loving adult self again, receiving a warm, wet, healthy baby girl into your own arms. Imagine what that feels like from the baby's experience—held and welcomed, thoroughly received, loved. Switch back and forth as much as you wish; this is your visualization. You have a right to go back in time and welcome your baby self into the world, healing any former trauma with your own comforting adult presence . . . letting yourself take full delight in all that felt good and pleasurable as you made your way down, imagining what it would have felt like to have experienced the pleasure of a healthy delivery with someone ready to love and hold you at birth.*

You may wish to have someone assist you, perhaps a friend or your partner. If you wish, ask this person to read the above exercise to you, perhaps even offering you comfort by holding your hand gently or touching you on your shoulder as you visualize your birth. This person needs only to be there for you. Only a loving, friendly presence is necessary to encourage you through this process.

It may be necessary to repeat the exercise several times in order to create a sensation of healthy, positive birth. If so, wait to repeat the exercise the following day. This will give your body a chance to integrate the new feeling. As you work through negative and painful associations of your own birth, whether they were brought to your awareness through family stories or from your own intuition, the visualization of a positive experience will come more easily. You have given your body a directive and permission to dream of new possibilities. This clears the way for you to associate positively to both your baby's reactions to being born and your own birth. The positive feelings that you imagine and daydream about provide your body with a new sensation.

Visualizations are like waking dreams; they link you to

your unconscious. In dreams your body experiences to some extent whatever you are dreaming. Patterns of sensation also occur in the body during visualization. Unlike a dream, however, visualization sends a conscious message to your unconscious. You consciously ask your unconscious to direct your imaginative energy toward a healthy delivery. In his book *The Psychobiology of Mind-Body Healing*, Ernest Rossi, Ph.D., shows that imagery is encoded neurochemically through the limbic-hypothalamic system of the brain. A compassionate visualization can help your body sense what a positive birth feels like.

After imagining what a safe and positive birth would be like from a baby's perspective, identify with it as fully as possible. Some women find it easy to do so, others must repeat the exercise several times. Whatever happens for you, do not judge yourself. Accept what comes as useful. Painful associations must be felt and healed before you can experience a new and enjoyable journey. Coming back to the exercise the following day can be surprisingly helpful —you will be able to proceed beyond any points that previously blocked your progress. Eventually the positive birthing visualization will be the one with which you identify. It will form a part of your foundation feelings, which are the unconscious associations and body memories that are activated as you approach labor. Healing any painful associations from your own birth liberates you from negative memory. The unconscious is then free to take on new and positive associations. Once you have been able to visualize a positive birth, write down the sensations that seemed important. These will be significant when you give birth, as the sensations will return to your consciousness and remind you how you want to welcome this baby to the world.

_____

_____

_____

_____

_____

_____

_____

_____

_____
_____
_____
_____
_____
_____
_____
_____
_____
_____
_____
_____

Did You Feel Loss or Neglect From Your Mother?

Pay attention to the feelings that arose about your own mother as you completed the exercise above. If feelings of neglect, loss, or emotional pain are a significant part of your relationship with your mother—whether in the present or the past—you may find that difficult associations or memories come up for healing now. If this is the case, be compassionate with yourself. Visualize your younger self at whatever age you were hurting (even if it was just yesterday) and offer your warmth and presence to her. Imagine yourself hugging or otherwise comforting this younger you. Mere acknowledgment of your past unmet needs will begin the healing process. You can do this exercise alone or in the presence of your partner or a supportive friend.

Mothers are not perfect human beings. If your own mother failed to support you in some essential way, it is now your responsibility to complete the mothering you missed, to meet your own needs. Giving to yourself in this way will provide you the energy and wholeness to give to your child. This exercise by no means encourages you to cast blame, as we all do the best job we possibly can with the resources we have available. You will make mistakes too. This exercise simply makes you a resource to yourself. Loving yourself is a prerequisite to nurturing another human being: Self-nurturance is a part of motherhood.

Now that you have reflected on your own birth, you are ready to turn your attention to any prior experience of childbirth. Clearing the way for a fresh start with your upcoming labor requires healing any unresolved emotional pain from an earlier childbirth. The transformation of negative experience—to any extent possible—will lead to greater peace and harmony as you approach your next labor.

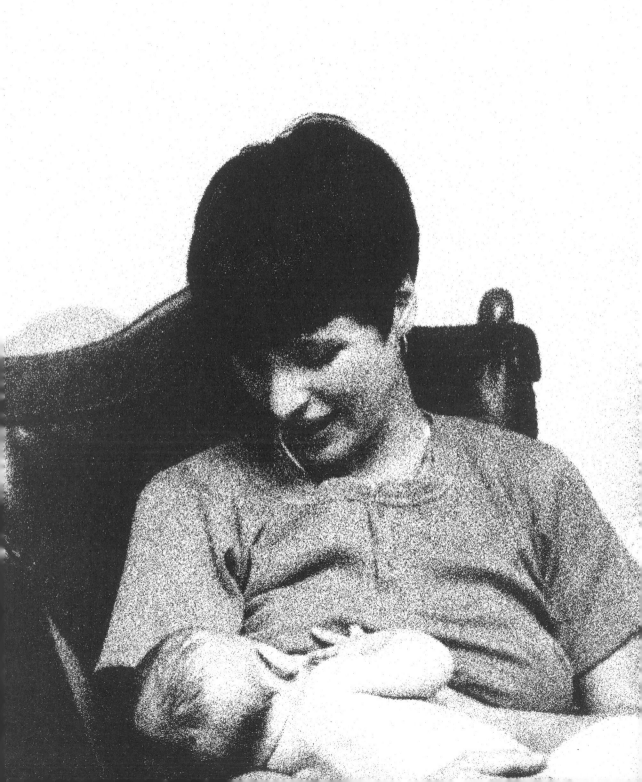

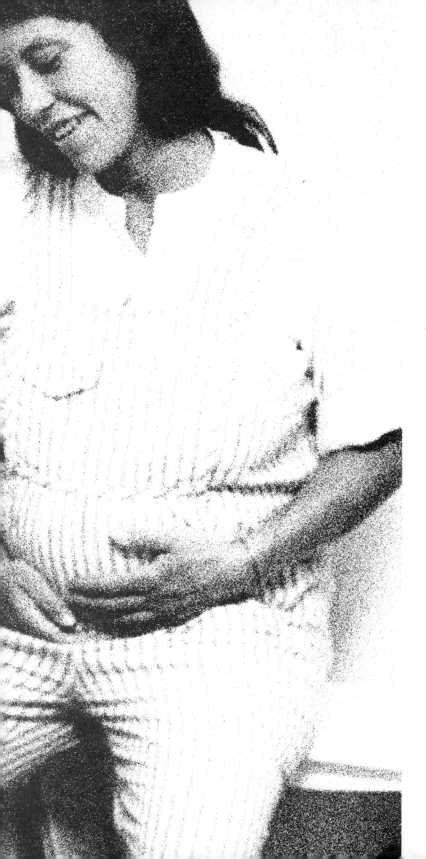

4

Previous Childbirth Experience and Cultural Messages

Past pregnancy and childbirth experiences lay the foundation for future births . . . along with cultural influences. . . .

CLAUDIA PANUTHOS
Transformation through Birth

THE SECOND WAY WE learn about birth is through our own childbearing. Prior impressions of childbirth are woven indelibly into our expectations for future labor. Giving birth is a powerful event that comes only a few times in the lives of most modern women. Whatever occurred during a previous birth is likely to be activated emotionally during the next. Working through your feelings about an earlier childbirth is an important part of preparing for your next. Flashbacks will influence your feelings during labor if you have not resolved emotionally charged memories.

If you already have been through a labor and childbirth that progressed smoothly, you have a body memory that will support you next time. Agreeable associations, particularly if the delivery was within four years, help you trust your body. Most women are assured and relaxed in a second childbirth if the first was a positive experience.

If, however, a woman had sufficient fear, perhaps because she was unprepared for labor or ill-equipped to deal with the pain of contractions, she may be left with a residue of anxiety that interferes with the next labor, even though the first birth was completely normal. If a previous childbirth was difficult due to complications of pregnancy or delivery, it becomes a part of a woman's emotional, and sometimes physical, body-learning for later childbirth. She may feel a lack of confidence in both her body and the labor process itself.

It is important to free yourself from former associations before labor begins again. The following examples show how a woman can identify with positive associations for a subsequent childbirth even though a previous one was complicated.

Linda, a thirty-six-year-old mother of five, came to see me because she had been induced for all her previous deliveries. She wondered if it might be possible to start labor spontaneously with her sixth. I discovered that although she had been through childbirth classes for each birth, she did not understand any of the theories on how labor begins. Her pregnancies continued one to two weeks past her due date each time. During her past three deliveries her water had broken but no labor ensued.

While she was in a relaxed state of light hypnosis, I explained to Linda how this time her baby might release a hormone that would stimulate her pituitary gland to release oxytocin, the hormone necessary to produce contractions. I also suggested that perhaps her other babies had released this hormone but her body had not responded to it for some reason. I assured her that in any case, her body could learn to recognize and respond to the early sensations of labor. I asked her to remember the contractions induced by the synthetic hormone Pitocin and to imagine her own body producing this feeling and starting labor on its own, at the right time for this baby. Indeed, with her sixth baby Linda's water broke and labor began. She gave birth for the first time with no induction of labor.

Linda had so identified with a belief in her body's inability to start labor that her heightened anxiety overrode any new expectations for labor. Her body may have been conditioned to an induced labor. Through deep relaxation she was able to visualize her water breaking and labor starting. Perhaps this helped her release tension that might otherwise have overridden her own hormones. Recent research on the role of the brain's limbic-hypothalamic system in hormone production and release supports this belief.

Other situations may be more complex. Cesarean birth may lead women to distrust their bodies, as may difficult vaginal delivery or loss of a baby through stillbirth, malformation, or other accidents of nature. Some women may have emotional associations that need clearing before they feel ready to give birth to another child. Such was the case with Anita.

Anita, then thirty years old, came to see me in the seventh month of her pregnancy. She was happily married and looking forward to motherhood. When Anita and her husband began to attend childbirth classes, however, she became distraught. Each time she tried to visualize herself in labor she became anxious and upset. Twelve years earlier she had delivered a baby that she gave up for adoption. Even though Anita had been anesthetized, had no memory of the delivery, and had never seen her child, her body remembered giving birth. Visualizing herself in labor, she previewed the feelings her body would remember when she again entered labor. During the first six months of pregnancy she had told herself repeatedly that this was really a first childbirth for her since she did not remember the other one. Indeed, she had wanted to forget that the first pregnancy had ever happened. Because of her intense guilt and sadness she felt unable to take advantage of her body's knowledge of childbirth. Instead she found herself increasingly disconnected from both her body and her baby.

Fortunately, she was able to address this disconnection before her next labor. With light hypnosis she was able to visualize being awake during her labor with her first child and holding her baby before she gave him to the nurse. Anita grieved the loss of her child and the sadness of her situation. She visualized talking with her baby, telling him why she had not been ready for motherhood or capable of caring for him. She forgave herself and began to realize that she had given him life and had mothered him by allowing him the opportunity to be loved and cared for by people who could do so. She began to appreciate herself for her courage and her body for having given birth.

By the following week Anita's anxiety was considerably diminished and she was able to visualize herself in labor with her present child. She gained assurance from the fact that her body had delivered a baby before. Anxiety no longer stood in the way of her body knowledge and her confidence in her body increased. By facing her emotional pain and accepting herself she was able to reconnect with the baby she carried. Having released the past she could make way for the future. She was able to visualize herself giving birth, a visualization that went as smoothly as did her four-hour labor with her second son.

Denying her past would have diverted Anita's energy during labor. She would have grappled with memories and ghosts, attempting to block out the labor process. By facing her fear she was able to regain her relationship with her body and to benefit from her body memory of childbirth.

If you have given birth before, write the story of your labor and delivery. Include any medical complications if they occurred, as well as your feelings at the time and your current feelings. You will bring associations with you to your next childbirth. By airing negative associations now, you will give yourself time to heal so that you can begin your next labor with a fresh outlook. Feelings that surface when your body approaches labor will be less likely to overwhelm you. You will not be surprised by ghosts from your past. Sad or frightening associations will lose their power to distort your present. They will retire to their rightful place in your past if given the chance to do so.

If your previous childbirth was a positive experience, write that in your story. Acknowledge the powerful resource of already having given birth.

Writing Your Childbirth Story

_____

_____

_____

_____

_____

_____

_____

_____

_____

_____

_____

_____

_____

_____

_____

_____

_____

_____

Now that you have written about your experience you may wish to share it with your partner or a friend. Keep in mind that whatever your experience of childbirth has been, it carries the seeds of a smoother journey for the next childbirth. By transforming any negative associations you are free to feel the positive resources you also have available.

Transforming Negative Experiences of Birth

Whatever your prior experience, there is always some positive gain for the body in learning how to give birth. If you once had a cesarean because you did not dilate more than five centimeters, you may feel your body failed. You may feel betrayed by your body and distrustful. It is also true, however, that your body stretched as it never had before and did, in fact, make it half-way to the full dilation needed to give birth. Remember that our bodies are always learning how to adjust and adapt to new situations. Women having first babies experience more complications because they have never given birth before. Statistically, second births are easier; the body has gained knowledge from the previous experience. If you dilated at all the first time, if the baby was delivered with such medical equipment as forceps or vacuum aspiration, if you did not have a labor but carried a baby to full term, even if there were complications at labor, your body has some knowledge of the process and is ready to learn more—if you give it the chance. There is much that your body did well.

Write down the ways your body did a good job for you. See if you can look at your former experience as a glass half full instead of half empty. This is closer to a true representation of what your body has done and can learn to do during your next labor. If, for example, you had a vaginal birth by forceps with your first baby, recognize that your first child paved the way for the next in many ways. He or she helped to open the passageway, and your body yielded. The next time you give birth you can remember that you stretched the passageway and thus garner the confidence, strength, and energy to push the second one through.

Remember that your body learns by doing. When you ride a bicycle, your body learns to adjust for balance. The first time you climb on, your body learns from doing. As time passes, you ride the bike easily; this knowledge is retained forever in your body. Riding is no longer something you think about; it is the result of an experiential learning that began with your initial attempt to ride, even though the first time you could not stay upright. Your body can use your earlier childbirth if anxiety doesn't block the learning process. Reframe your experience, highlighting the aspects that might aid you during your next childbirth. *Reframing*, in this context, means acknowledging the experience you had in the past for its potential positive impact on the future.

_____

_____

_____

_____

_____

_____

_____

_____

_____

_____

_____

_____

_____

_____

Healing Previous Birth Experiences

The following passage can be read aloud by a friend or your partner while you close your eyes and visualize. You may also choose to read it into a tape recorder and play it back to yourself. Or you may choose to read it through once, then slowly again as you take time to visualize between sentences.

Take a few minutes to recall the childbirth that you want to heal. Remember what you were wearing at the time you went into labor. Who was with you? What were the surroundings like? Imagine that you can take an older and wiser you back to the side of your younger self in labor. Visualize the older and wiser you being there to comfort your younger self. Imagine you can hold her with all the love and compassion you have ever given to anyone. Give it to her now. Speak directly to the younger self now, telling her anything she needed to hear back then. Was there anything the younger you would have liked to have said back then, but didn't? Listen to her tell you what she needs.

Imagine that there is some resource she needed then that you can give to her now. Imagine giving her that resource. Perhaps it was strength, courage, acceptance, love, or anything else she needed. See her absorb that resource and watch her change in some subtle but important way. See her absorb what she needs in order to heal, to make her feel whole.

With compassion, hold her in your arms. Comfort her. Then bring her back with you, slowly, lovingly, through time. And feel her whole, healed. After you have sensed her wholeness, bring yourself back to this room and to your present surroundings. Take your time to come back to your environment.

It is often the case that having lived through a trauma, we will push away the part of ourselves that experienced the pain. Psychologists have labeled this dissociation *psychic numbing.* This can cause yet another emotional wounding because we are rejecting ourselves. Initially this disconnection may be necessary; your psyche seeks to shield you from pain. Later, however, it can create difficulty. Such was the case with Anita, who experienced disconnection from both her body and her unborn baby because she refused to feel the loss of her first child. Self-acceptance is the cure for feelings of self-blame or rejection, which are so often the result of a frightening experience. Reconnecting with this past self before your next delivery can help. You will find new energy available as this lost part of yourself finds its way home.

In the unlikely event that feelings of being frightened or overwhelmed persist, seek help from a qualified counselor or psychotherapist. Dealing with these feelings now will allow you to relax during your next labor.

Birth: An Opportunity for Learning

Giving birth opens doors—to our own resources as well as to a new life. Maturity comes as we deal with difficulties on life's path. Our personalities become more defined as we face challenges. Always, birth provides us with an opportunity for learning. Even in very difficult circumstances we often have more choices than we imagine we have. In childbirth, as in other life events, it is important to hear what others have learned. Anne's struggle to overcome the fearful memories of her first child's premature delivery offers a good lesson.

Anne's daughter was delivered by cesarean section. The baby had a rare pancreatic disorder, which required immediate surgery. Until the baby began to thrive one month after birth, Anne feared losing her infant. During her second pregnancy, Anne was bombarded with nightmarish memories of her daughter's birth. Told that her daughter's illness might have been genetic, she struggled against her expectations for the worst. She faced her terror of once again going through a life-threatening scenario. During this process she learned more about herself and the choices she had in the present. The following is her answer to the anxiety she faced in her second pregnancy:

The only thing I can do, that I have the most input into, is to enjoy this pregnancy. I realize that I can either reach the end of this pregnancy with whatever it brings, having enjoyed and received energy from the pregnancy . . . or I can reach the end of my pregnancy drained, having spent the entire time afraid. . . . Going into labor, facing new motherhood, taking care of a brand new baby, with special needs or not . . . I have to give myself this gift of renewal to do the work ahead. It is the only thing I have input into.

The only gift I can give myself is to enjoy this pregnancy. . . . Because I can't give myself answers about what happened the last time. But I can give myself whatever strength, joy, and renewal I can get out of this pregnancy. Many times I have felt terrified and afraid . . . but this [gift of renewal] has been my link, my key, to flow through my pregnancy.

Anne reported feeling a calm unlike any she ever had before, even during her first pregnancy, even before anything frightening had ever happened to her. Facing the terror gave her new resources for living and especially for dealing with her next childbirth. Indeed, she was able to give birth to her second child with a vaginal delivery. Acknowledging fear can deepen our reserves and help us discover fresh meaning and commitment in our lives. Birth is literally the threshold of life, a doorway that is also an opening to psychological growth and a deeper knowledge of our physical selves. Do not judge your fear or anxiety. Confront and befriend the fear, and it will yield an inner treasure. Emotional and psychological pressures in life serve to facilitate new learning and development.

Is there anything you learned about yourself from your last childbirth that opened you to yourself or life in a deeper way? Is anything changing for you now as you approach your next labor and new motherhood? Write down any new insights that come to mind, any thoughts, feelings, or reflections on your past childbirth and what it taught you about yourself. If you did not like what happened, did you learn anything that can help you next time? What can you do that will make a difference now? Challenge yourself to identify some feeling, attitude, or belief that you can explore and that will help you as you approach your next labor.

_____

_____

_____

_____

_____

_____

_____

_____

_____

_____

_____

_____

_____

_____

_____

_____

_____

_____

Releasing Anger The following exercises will help you complete your healing process, especially if you have negative feelings about your medical treatment or anger at particular people involved in the childbirth.

If you had complications during childbirth, you may feel angry as well as sad. Some women feel as though they have been robbed and don't know why. You may have a great relationship with your baby now and be entirely content with motherhood and your new family yet still feel upset about what happened to you during labor. If this is the case for you, be aware that these are normal feelings. Childbirth is a rite of passage for women, and oftentimes medical professionals, partners, or other family members may not understand why a woman feels cheated. After all, she has a normal healthy baby, doesn't she? Not having her feelings taken seriously can contribute to vague feelings of inadequacy or even postpartum depression. It is important to express your sadness and anger.

If you find yourself with unexpressed or unresolved anger about your past childbirth, try to make appointments to talk with the people who provided care during your earlier disappointing childbirth. Express your feelings and ask questions that remain unanswered. There are times when medical personnel have been insensitive or unresponsive because of overly busy schedules or an inability to understand the emotional dimensions of the childbirth event. It is possible that misunderstandings can be bridged even after the fact.

If this is not possible or desirable, or if you feel it is more important to acknowledge your feelings to yourself than to confront someone else about them, then imagine you are having a discussion with the people involved. Whether medical personnel or family members, they may be people you feared in some way. If you felt betrayed by your doctor, you may have chosen another doctor but not given yourself the chance to trust him or her. If you were angry at a nurse, you may not be able to establish the kind of relationship you will need with your next labor-and-delivery nurse. If anger at past care givers keeps you from communicating with or establishing trust in your current physician or midwife, then you are being haunted.

The best way to chase out the ghosts that are following you is to turn around and speak directly to them. Imagine exactly what you would say to these people if you felt safe enough to do so. Tell them how you felt, what you needed. In your fantasy, watch as the person listens to you with respect. Express your feelings fully. When you have finished, have the ghost ask you what you need to hear now, how she or he can answer your present needs. Perhaps an acknowledgment, an apology—or simply an understanding that was not expressed. Do not engage in arguments or dialogue that leads you away from this outcome. This is your visualization. You can imagine whatever you would like to hear.

You can also do this exercise with a friend or partner for support. Or you may wish to have the other person role-play the so-called ghost. Give this person instructions to listen respectfully, reflect understanding of your feelings, apologize, and do whatever else you require.

**Visualizing
a Positive Experience**

After you have confronted any ghosts from your past, allow yourself to relax. Imagine what it would have felt like to have given birth as you had wished—for example, vaginally, with love and support, and without complications.

Imagine as fully as you can what it would have felt like to have your baby come right down and through your vagina, with a strong heartbeat. You are pushing, your baby begins to crown, you can feel a burning sensation as you pant and begin to stretch around your baby's head—and here comes your baby, right out of your vagina, born healthy and handed into your arms. Or maybe you reach for your baby yourself, gently guiding it into the world.

Watch this new image as if it were an alternate memory, sort of a movie in your mind. Imagining it can help you heal some of what might have been hurting, but more importantly the image can give you a sense of the normal process. Your body registers the sensation of what you imagine deeply, it creates a memory tracing of your visualization. You are communicating to your body consciousness your desire to adjust and adapt to your next labor.

Complete the exercise by sending loving energy to yourself. Addressing yourself by name, say: "I love you, _____." Although it may feel a bit silly at first, you will find that directing love to yourself verbally, just as you do to other people, has a profound impact. It is common for embarrassment to dissolve into loving tears when you finally reach yourself with your own words. Repeat the phrase several times to yourself, until you can absorb the message.

Again, if you wish, you may ask a partner or friend to be present with you or read some of the above exercise to you while you close your eyes and imagine. You may want to do this exercise two or three times over a one-week period. This gives your unconscious mind a chance to play with the movie, and you might find it much easier to imagine the second or third time you try it. Like learning how to ride a bicycle, your unconscious learnings take practice and time.

We are especially influenced by relatives' stories, particularly if they come from women with whom we identify. Movies and television shows about birth may also teach us emotional attitudes and expectations. When there is no other context in which to learn about childbirth, young girls, in particular, may be susceptible to media messages —whether of strength and joy or of helplessness and danger. These messages can become a script about birth that is stored in the emotional center of a child's brain.

Cultural Messages That Influence Childbirth

Because birth has been removed from the home and institutionalized, few first-time mothers have any direct experience with childbirth. Prior to the 1970s most hospitals did not permit family members to participate in or even witness another family member's birth. Mommy disappeared into the hospital and emerged with an infant. Stories and jokes about taking the baby back to the hospital seemed real to children who believed that the hospital had given the baby to the mother. Childbirth was a shrouded subject, so women did not learn the skills needed to cope with a natural birth. Even today, few know what to expect in a normal labor. Unable to gain this knowledge directly, most young girls look to movies or soap operas for the story of childbirth.

The film versions of birth carry much greater impact when there is no real, first-hand knowledge available. Unfortunately, normal birth makes a less dramatic script than women delivering unassisted in elevators, dying in childbirth, or enduring rare complications. The message young girls hear is often one of danger, weakness, and fear rather than strength and empowerment. Even when relatively benign, the media's description of the childbirth process is usually indirect and unrealistic.

Many women were not even told about how their mothers experienced childbirth. Others heard nightmarish tales of intervention and isolation. Some mothers simply refused to tell their daughters anything because they themselves wanted to forget, and silence was protection. Other mothers felt they had little to teach their daughters, and besides, the young women would soon discover for themselves. Descriptions, when given, were often kept short and simple. *You gave me a difficult time,* might have been a mother's only comment to her daughter. The physical details of birth were seldom discussed, and few women learned anything about the real process from their own mothers.

Messages of Strength, Yielding, and Dependency

The dominant cultural message, whether from television, film, or literature, has been that women are weak and need men to take care of them. Of course, this is not necessarily what women learn in their homes. Ethnic or family patterns may amplify or modify this message. Nevertheless, our culture affects our biology; women who have been taught that they are only fragile and delicate will experience dissonance when they look to themselves for the strength needed during the intense work of labor.

The women's movement has fought this cultural message of weakness and inferiority. Each wave of feminism has sought to restore power by proclaiming women's strength and equality. By the early 1970s women were educating themselves about their bodies. The Boston Women's Health Collective published *Our Bodies, Ourselves*, which encouraged women to empower themselves in all aspects of health care, including childbirth.

Childbirth requires women to develop their feminine power, a strength that is akin to the nature of water: yielding but relentless.

Self-Reliance and Dependency

Labor requires women to depend on others, just as some species of dolphins may rely on another dolphin to help bring their babies to the ocean's surface for their first breath. Dependency makes us vulnerable, however, so it is often confused with weakness. In the early phase of the women's movement, dependency was feared and sometimes scorned. Yet in labor a woman needs support. This is not weakness; it is part of being human.

Pregnancy and labor are periods of vulnerability. This vulnerability is not weakness but softness, which later contributes to adjustment to motherhood. Feeling dependent may open you to your need for help, and the ability to accept help from others can increase your strength and endurance for labor. Each of us must come to terms with our own feminine strength and our need for protection. Perhaps the story of Hanna will help you in your own struggle to integrate the culture's contradictory messages about women and power.

Hanna was single and expecting her first child. She perceived herself as a strong woman, and indeed she was. She ran marathons, lifted weights, and cycled long distances. Despite her strong physique she was frustrated by labor. All she could do was wait and breathe through the contractions until she reached full dilation. She was irritated with this passivity and overjoyed when she could finally push. She pushed so hard and with such tremendous force that her cervix began to swell. She quickly exhausted herself with her efforts. Her contractions became ineffective and her baby began to retreat instead of descend into the vagina.

Having focused on her need to be strong, Hanna could not cope with the ebb and flow of labor. She couldn't see that yielding and accepting support from others are positive, active forces. She had mistaken yielding and the human need for support as weakness.

Hanna had to be convinced by her close female friend that she could not push the baby out in one gigantic effort of will and physical power. She was instructed by her doctor to let her friends hold her, to release her body weight into their arms. As her baby descended, she learned how to yield to her contractions, to soften her strength. She also learned to depend on others to help her, to trust her friends to give her emotional and physical support. After the birth she joked that she finally understood the wise old saying, You cannot push the river, it flows by itself. Hanna had learned to yield to the birth force flowing through her.

Women feel conflicted as they grapple with the dichotomy between vulnerability and strength. Coming to terms with femininity in our culture is a challenge. Hanna exemplifies the struggle to balance the need for support from others with the equally important need for self-reliance. As you go through labor, you will develop your own femininity while contributing to the collective female experience. Whatever your journey, it is important to the generations of women who will follow. Giving birth requires both strength and yielding—the ability to be both self-reliant and willing to depend on others for loving support. This balance integrates the contradictory messages of our culture. It is the acceptance of interdependence that allows you to create a healthy balance in your relationships.

Childbirth Education: A Medical Mystique

Further confusion about the childbirth process came from the medical world. Led by male experts in the field, obstetricians and childbirth educators attempted to help women develop positive attitudes toward childbirth by down-playing the pain of labor. In the 1940s English obstetrician Grantly Dick-Read hypothesized that women feel pain during labor because they are afraid. His book *Childbirth without Fear* helped popularize the notion of natural childbirth.

French obstetrician Fernand Lamaze encouraged women to believe that labor could be managed so that it would not be painful. His techniques for relaxation and breathing, presented in his popular book *Painless Childbirth*, are still used. In an era when most were still "knocked out with medication" for their baby's arrival, Lamaze helped many women be conscious and present with their babies immediately after delivery. Statistics on the effects of his method for reducing pain and the need for medication during labor were inconclusive, but clearly his method was not as successful as its popularity would suggest.

American obstetrician Robert Bradley's method of husband-coached childbirth also focused on relaxation and added the element of support from the partner. But Bradley's techniques, popularized in the early 1960s, still failed to prepare women for the pain of labor.

Social anthropologist Sheila Kitzinger's book *The Experience of Childbirth*, published in 1962, encouraged women to listen to their bodies and to surrender to the flow of birth rather than adhering to disciplined breathing methods that separated them from the experience. Kitzinger successfully communicated the depth and richness of the emotional aspects of pregnancy and birth. But it wasn't until 1981 that the concept of healthy pain was brought to the attention of childbirth educators; in my book *Birthing Normally*, I described my success with a method of body-centered childbirth preparation that confronted the issue of pain directly.

Doing research for the book, I attended a large number of births, both in private homes and at hospitals. I observed that techniques being taught in childbirth classes did not offer realistic preparation for labor. I felt that women were not emotionally ready for the reality of pain, and that this hindered both their physiological labor and their ability to cope—and I believed that the two were related. I felt that preparation with body-centered methods rather than those that encouraged dissociation from the body would help women to integrate the experience beforehand. My belief in the effectiveness of a body-centered method was supported by a three-year study at the Berkeley Family Health Center in California. Between 1977 and 1980, 350 women— 80 percent having first babies—were prepared by my method. For purposes of the study, the women were considered medication-free if they did not request or receive medication for pain at any time during labor for a vaginal birth or any time prior to a cesarean section if it occurred. Only five of these women needed pain medication during labor. It wasn't until I researched the effectiveness of other methods of preparation that I discovered that the body-centered approach had been more successful in helping women achieve unmedicated childbirth than had other methods previously available in Western society.

When women are not given techniques to cope with normal pain, they may believe something is going wrong in the labor. Some women have reported to me that when they felt pain they thought they were not breathing correctly or relaxing enough. Many withdrew from the process in shame and confusion. Fear that something is wrong or feelings of self-blame distract women from the need to cope with contractions as they come.

Perhaps it took the years since natural childbirth was first embraced by Grantly Dick-Read in the 1940s for childbirth education to transcend our old cultural standards of ladylike behavior. If women were to give birth naturally in a hospital it was important that they be in control, which some interpreted as being quiet and not disturbing others. Women were not prepared or encouraged to lose their inhibitions during labor. But being a hostess to others while simultaneously coping with labor is a difficult, if not impossible, task.

Hospital procedures have changed dramatically in the last twenty years, as have many of our social norms. Women are now freer to express themselves. Nevertheless, pressure to be ladylike can still suppress a woman's natural means of coping with labor. An inability to cope effectively can lead to anxiety, fear, and disruptions in the labor process.

Demystifying Childbirth   Removing birth from the home setting and family members during the first half of the twentieth century created a cultural mystique of childbirth that affected women's ability to prepare for labor. This mystification spread throughout the culture, from movies to sex education. When women were finally ready to reclaim their rights to natural, family-centered birth, they were left with little firsthand knowledge of the process itself. To some extent childbirth education set women up for failure by not confronting the issue of pain directly.

The next three chapters will address common misconceptions about labor and offer methods for realistic preparation. In chapter 5 you will find exercises that foster a realistic understanding of the emotional and physical experience of childbirth. It is important for couples to increase communication in preparation for labor, and the exercises in chapter 6 will help you do this. Chapter 6 also has guidelines for having your other children attend the birth. Exercises for coping with the normal pain and intensity of childbirth are described in chapter 7. Women prepared through this body-centered method show a striking decrease in need for medication during labor.

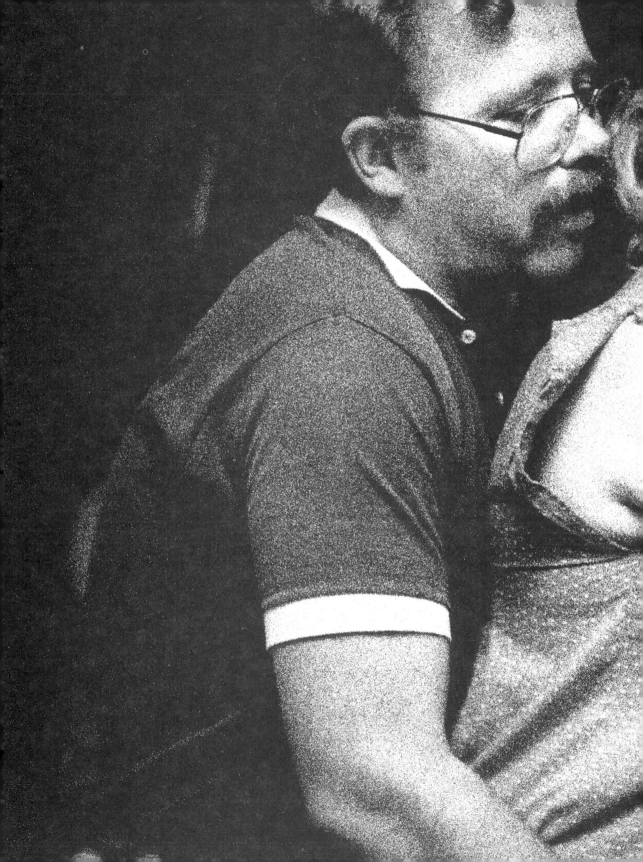

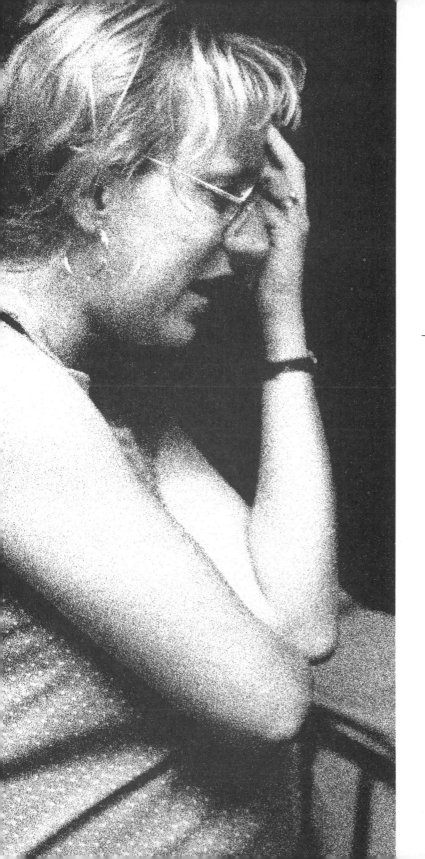

5

Preparing for Labor

It is not 'ladylike' to give birth. The strength and power of labor is not demure.

RHONDA
midwife

ANXIETY ABOUT THE UNKNOWN is common, as is excitement, especially for first-time mothers. Although we all know that millions upon billions of women have given birth before, we do not know what the experience will be like for us. Birth is universal yet it remains a mystery. Like love, labor is difficult to describe in words. It is the work of each pregnant woman to seek a personal understanding of the process of childbirth.

The Stages of Labor Labor is a progression of energy outward, culminating in your baby's birth. Like pregnancy, it builds. For medical purposes, labor is described as consisting of three stages. While it is useful to know the broad definitions of these stages, it is also important to understand that these divisions are artificial—a scientific attempt to label nature's mystery.

Doctors measure first-stage labor by the dilation of the cervix from zero to ten centimeters. This stage has two distinct phases: early and active labor. They represent the longest part of the process and will be discussed in detail.

Second-stage labor is the baby's descent through the birth canal and into the world. Since the second stage is measured medically from the time of full dilation, not from the engagement of the baby's head in the pelvis, it can take from twenty minutes to several hours. This stage averages sixty to ninety minutes for first babies but depends on the baby's placement in the pelvis when the cervix is fully dilated. If the baby is still high in the pelvis, it may take longer to descend; if the baby is low, the second stage may be shorter. In her book *Childbirth with Insight*, physical therapist Elizabeth Noble says the second stage might be managed better if it were measured from the time a woman feels the urge to push. She suggests that this urge comes when the baby is low enough to stimulate nerve endings in the bottom of the pelvis (pelvic floor), which then carry a message to the pituitary gland to release more oxytocin, a hormone that causes labor contractions. Some mothers, however, never feel an urge to push. Their sensation is one of increasingly intense contractions as the baby eases its way through the vagina.

The third stage of labor begins after the delivery of the

baby. As the uterus contracts down to its prepregnant size, the placenta separates naturally. When the placenta is expelled, usually within twenty minutes after birth, labor is complete.

First-time mothers may be surprised to feel Braxton-Hicks contractions—named after the physician who first described them—which usually occur in the last six weeks of pregnancy. If you have already had a baby, you may notice these painless contractions as early as your fifth month of pregnancy. Braxton-Hicks contractions do not dilate the cervix. You might think of these gentle tightenings as your uterus's rehearsal for labor.

Although no one knows exactly what triggers labor, some researchers believe that the baby releases a hormone that stimulates the mother's pituitary gland to secrete oxytocin. Even before these contractions begin, your own hormonal changes at the end of pregnancy may have softened the cervix. Signs that labor is imminent include the show of blood as the mucus plug that seals the cervix is lost and leakage of water—the amniotic fluid surrounding your baby.

When your baby is ready to be born, the cervix gradually begins to change. As it softens, it yields to the pressure of your baby's head. Some nurse midwives, among them Paula Holtz of Santa Cruz, California, believe that the baby helps labor through a reflex in which it pushes its feet against the hardened uterus, burrowing its head deeper into your pelvis. The baby and the uterine contractions work together to apply pressure to the softening cervix, which dilates to ten centimeters, or five fingers, in diameter. With the continuing momentum of contractions, your baby makes headway through the cervix, into the birth canal, finally emerging at the vaginal opening. Reaching for your baby at the moment of birth, seeing his or her face, smelling your baby's skin, and hearing the first cry are all experiences that await you.

Second and subsequent labors generally progress at about twice the speed of a first labor—sometimes faster. In the medical textbook *Obstetrics and Gynecology*, the authors note that length of labor is affected by many factors (italics added):

The duration of labor in any given individual is determined by her parity, the size and position of the baby, the capacity of the pelvis, the consistency of the cervix, the efficiency of the uterine mechanism [contractions], and *the patient's attitude toward pregnancy and womanhood.*

Since so many factors contribute to the duration of labor, it is important to follow your body's lead rather than cling tightly to preconceived expectations.

Early Labor:
The Misunderstood Stage

The first stage is the most misunderstood part of labor. Ignorance about what to expect may lead to premature exhaustion and protracted labor. It is important to understand that early labor is different from active labor.

The beginning of labor is slow and gradual. Early labor, the softening and initial opening of the cervix, may occur days or even weeks before active labor begins. The average first-time mother experiences one to two days of early labor as contractions come and go, often irregularly. In the first stage of labor the hormonal changes usually take effect slowly. The cervix dilates the first couple of centimeters more slowly than it does as labor progresses.

In early labor, contractions may slow down or spontaneously disappear during sleep or physical activity. Or, contractions may continue regularly throughout the day. Some blood-tinged mucus may appear as the cervix begins to soften and open. It may be a full day until you are actually in active labor. When you are, contractions may intensify, instead of stopping, with sleep or physical activity.

You will find techniques for coping with the pain of active labor in chapter 7. Your first preparation, however, will be to learn the difference between the early and active phases. Active labor generally begins when the cervix has dilated between three to four centimeters for a first baby and about four to five for subsequent labors. These are approximate figures and may vary. There is a point, however, when the cervix is stretched far enough that the pressure of the baby's head and the force of the contractions will increase labor's momentum.

When the cervix has softened and opened this wide, little

resistance remains to complete dilation. After this point the cervix dilates approximately one centimeter per hour, meaning it will usually take another six to eight hours to complete dilation, or ten centimeters. Variations are normal, but it is important to get a sense of the average labor and what you might expect. You can then adjust to your body's unique labor rhythm.

First-time mothers are seldom taught the demarcation between the early (sometimes referred to as latent) and active phases of first-stage labor. If this is your first baby, you should expect the early phase to last from one to two days before active labor ensues.

Consult with your prenatal care provider when you are deciding where to spend your time during early labor. Some women planning to give birth in a hospital will remain home, in close contact with their doctor or midwife, until they reach active labor. Talk with your practitioner about the best time for going to the hospital. Some physicians and midwives will ask you to come to the office during early labor so they can check your dilation and the baby's heartbeat. This will help them determine the best time to settle you into the hospital or for them to come to the house if you are planning a home birth.

First-Stage Labor: Early and Active Phases

The best way to deal with the early phase of first-stage labor is generally to go about your usual activities as much as possible. Usually contractions consume all your attention and draw you inward, even during early labor. If you haven't experienced labor previously, you will tend to believe that your labor is further along that it actually is. If so, you are vulnerable to letting your mind jump far ahead of your body. When this happens, some women stop eating or sleeping because they are excited and believe themselves to be in labor. They are, of course, but usually it is only early labor.

What I call the beached-whale syndrome occurs when a women uses up all her resources early in her labor. She doesn't get the sleep, rest, or food that she needs, resulting in total exhaustion by the time she reaches the active phase. This is unfortunate because it isn't until late in labor when she needs to exert energy for pushing. When she finally does progress to the second stage, she may lack the strength to push her baby out. By then she may be so depleted she requires medical intervention.

Focusing Your Attention during Early Labor

You need to understand clearly when you are in the early phase. If you put your concentration elsewhere between contractions, you will eventually be led into active labor by your body at about three to four centimeters dilation.

You will find that when you are indeed in active labor, you will be less able to put your concentration outside yourself between contractions. The transition from early to active labor is marked by a change in the quality of your consciousness and your ability to concentrate. Projects that keep you focused outside yourself provide you with a way to monitor this. Activities such as baking a pie, knitting a sweater, or playing a parlor game focus your attention outward. Your inability to do so between contractions help you discriminate early labor from active labor.

Most women find it more comfortable to stay at home during early labor and unless there is medical indication otherwise, physicians and midwives generally encourage mothers to do just that. If there is any possibility that you might find yourself laboring in the hospital before you are three centimeters dilated, it is a good idea to bring early-labor projects with you. They will engage your attention between contractions until you are further dilated.

Some women need medical supervision even during early labor, others simply feel more comfortable getting situated in the place they will be delivering. If either is the case for you, follow your needs but do not mistake going to the hospital for making the baby come faster.

In the early phase, labor is impressionable: When you change your environment contractions may slow or even stop. When active labor has begun, however, you will find that your body's response to change of environment will be an increase rather than a decrease in the strength of contractions. The completion of delivery has become the body's command, regardless of outside disruptions. This is nature's way. When you are in active labor, your body tends to stimulate the labor process rather than inhibit its force. In the early phase, your labor is more easily interrupted, so it's a good idea to wait until your labor is in full swing before going to the hospital.

As you progress into active labor you will be settling into the environment in which you have chosen to give birth. A place where you feel safe and supported provides you with the best opportunity for releasing fear and enjoying the comforting hands and voices of those around you.

Remain in contact with your medical care givers. If you are delivering in a hospital, they can help you decide when to go there. You may wish to be checked for dilation by your doctor or midwife before admitance to the hospital. If you are remaining at home, your midwife or doctor will usually come to your home when you can no longer talk on the phone between contractions. The women's inability to conduct a phone conversation has long been a sign for home-birth practitioners dealing with first-time mothers; they recognize it as a signal that the laboring woman is in active labor.

When you begin feeling tightening of your uterus during the last several weeks of pregnancy, you may in fact be in the very early phase of labor. While they are not dilating the cervix, these Braxton-Hicks contractions may be helping to soften your cervix at this time.

As you get closer to your due date you may feel minor cramping with these uterine tightenings. Contractions may build as they begin to soften, then dilate your cervix. As these contractions get stronger and more consistent during early labor you will find that they increase with physical activity. Walking or bending over may bring on further contractions instead of inhibiting them as might have been the case earlier.

Whether or not you ask your practitioner to check for dilation at this time is usually your decision.

If you are checked for dilation, your doctor or midwife may inform you that you are a certain percentage effaced and a fingertip or more dilated. Effacement is a term used when calculating the softening of the cervix. The cervix shortens and softens prior to, and simultaneous with, dilation. This is called cervical effacement.

By the time contractions are coming regularly, you may

want to put your attention on projects that will take your focus away from labor while you are between contractions.

While you are having contractions, of course, you will need to stop what you are doing and focus your attention inward. Breathe, breathe, breathe. This is your only job at this time. Listen to your breath until the contraction fades away. Then return your attention to your previous activity.

Activities such as making bread from scratch, gardening, reading or being read to by your partner, playing a game of chess, Scrabble, or cards, or anything else that will occupy your attention externally can be used as an early-labor project. Your partner can assist you by reminding you to turn your attention toward this activity between contractions. You will find that during early labor you can engage yourself in an activity if you try. You may even feel quite normal and like your usual self while you are doing these activities. When the next contraction comes, however, you will have to stop whatever it is you are doing and focus on slow, deep breathing as the contraction moves through you.

A contraction is a very powerful sensation, even during early labor, and it requires your attention. For a first baby, you will find that even early-labor contractions are all-consuming while they are happening. Yet when the contraction is over, your attention can return to external activities. By returning to early-labor projects between contractions you are less likely to fall into the beached-whale syndrome described earlier. Without planning for this external focus, however, first-time mothers and their partners almost inevitably waste precious energy. If you match your expectation to the process, you will experience a smoother labor.

I encourage women to refrain from defining themselves as in labor until they reach the active phase. Women using my approach perceive themselves as having shorter labors, as they do not begin watching the clock until then.

Early-Labor Projects   Write down at least five activities that might serve as early-labor projects. Discuss these with your partner or labor coach and be certain that he or she understands the purpose of these activities. This person can help by reminding you to return to the project between contractions.

_____

_____

_____

_____

_____

_____

   Generally you are in active labor when you can no longer
return to your early-labor activity between contractions. It
is important that you be reminded to return your attention
to your activity and that you attempt to do so, thus giving
yourself a chance to break the spell of the contraction on
your conscious mind. This way it will be more likely that
your body leads you into labor, instead of your mind jump-
ing ahead of the process.

   Your early-labor project will help you stay aware of the
quality of your attention between contractions. Your level
of attention serves as an internal signal of where you are
in labor. You will find it a more effective guideline than
reliance on the clock.

Women are often taught to estimate labor's progress by
the minutes between contractions. The expectation is that
the time between contractions will consistently shorten and
that when they are three minutes apart you are in active
labor. This expectation can be misleading.

Time and Labor

   Sometimes, labor progresses consistently, with contractions remaining five minutes apart. Conversely, some
women have contractions three minutes apart from the
beginning of early labor. Focusing attention on time is a
cognitive, or left brain, approach to labor. It does not alert
you to an internal signal as does the technique of focusing
on early-labor projects.

   Labor is an experiential process best approached from
a right-hemisphere perspective—one that puts you in
touch with what is happening in your body. The right
hemisphere is also the part of the brain stimulated by relaxation and imagery, such as the birth visualization exercise described in chapter 8. By engaging in early-labor
projects you allow your interest to be absorbed. Labor pro-

gresses without mental interference. Similarly, we have all observed how interminable time feels when we are waiting and watching for a large pot of water to boil. As we turn our attention to other activities in the kitchen, we are soon, it seems, drawn back to the pot by the sound of the bubbling water.

Letting Go of Control

Labor requires that you yield rather than take control. Taking control of labor is the role of the physician in times of distress or abnormality. In a normal course of labor, a woman must react to the energy traveling through her. Her response is akin to moving with an ocean wave, sensing the flexible nature of the water as it changes its shape, flowing around the contours of land and shore. Following the natural flow of contractions allows you to cooperate with the force of nature.

Give yourself permission to express yourself during labor. Whether it's yelling through a contraction, complaining, grunting, or cursing, each woman must find her way of releasing tension. This release is a far more important goal than complete relaxation during contractions. Finding ways to express and release tension during contractions will ensure that you can relax and rest more completely between them.

Working through labor contractions is a little like mountain climbing. Your muscles strain as you pull yourself upward, then you rest between efforts—perhaps unsure if you ever want to do this again. But when you finally reach the mountaintop and look out over the valleys and sky, your awareness of having climbed there rewards you with a triumph you wouldn't feel if you had been deposited there by helicopter. As you meet your baby at the end of labor, you will feel this reward. We must trust that nature has its purpose in introducing us to our newborns after a period of hard work. Part of the intensity of labor comes from the physiological opening of the cervix to ten centimeters, which happens only when giving birth. There is also a simultaneous psychological and emotional intensity to labor that may facilitate bonding in the moments immediately following delivery. Meeting your baby at the peak of this concentration, when everything else fades away, may heighten your response.

The only breathing you will need to do during most of your labor is a natural extension of normal breathing. Slow, deliberate, and steady breaths through each contraction ensure that you and your baby receive the necessary oxygen. Four to five breaths (seven seconds for each inhalation and each exhalation) is an average number per contraction, however the most important thing is that you keep oxygen moving through you. As labor progresses your breathing requires more of your attention. Vocalization during active labor is a natural extension of breathing and serves to release tension caused by pain.

Breathing through Labor

You should be able to hear your own breath during contractions so that you can use the sound as a reassurance that you are not holding your breath. Avoid breath holding during the first stage of labor. Many people cease breathing as an instinctive response to pain. You can overcome this response simply by listening to your breath through each contraction. This is the single most important guideline for labor.

When your midwife or doctor tells you that your cervix is fully dilated, you have entered the second stage of labor. For some women the second stage may feel like a relief, as they are able to take a more active role in the process. Most women, however, do not experience any great change—just increasing intensity until the baby is born. This is an important point as some women are lulled into thinking that when dilation is complete, their labor is nearly over or their work is almost done. This misunderstanding does not prepare them to finish labor. It serves women better simply to prepare for a continuation of the process into the second stage. Increased vocalization is a common way of coping with this stage of labor. It encourages a release of tension and can effectively engage the diaphragm to help push the baby out.

Second-Stage Breathing

Occasionally, when the time comes to push, a woman discovers that she pushes more effectively if she holds her breath. This is the exception. Most women adjust to pushing by continuing the natural deep breathing that was used for first-stage labor. More often than not, this deep breathing progresses to vocalizing as you push your baby through your vagina during the second stage.

If there is little or no result from your pushing, you may find that holding your breath during a contraction is effective. Ask your doctor or midwife for feedback about the baby's descent. Usually you will find that grunting, or yelling, or other forms of vocalization are useful releases and help you to push naturally and instinctively. Use your labor attendants to help you determine the most effective pushing style for you. Remember, however, that labor is a continuous progression, which may not require any changes in how you are coping already.

Crowning and Birth   When your baby crowns, birth is imminent. Crowning refers to the point in labor when the baby's head is not only visible during contractions, but remains visible and no longer slides back between contractions. As the baby travels through the vagina, it surges forward with a contraction, then retreats slightly. This allows your vaginal opening to stretch and adapt to the circumference of your baby's head. It will only be another one or two contractions until your baby's head emerges! Many times, it will take another full contraction for your baby to turn its shoulders as it accommodates your pelvic bone. Occasionally a third contraction is needed for the rest of the baby's body to be born.

From the point of crowning you will begin to feel a burning sensation as the baby fully stretches your vagina. At this time, it is important that you not add to the pressure by pushing with a contraction. Instead, lessen the pressure by using a panting breath through these final contractions. This is the only time to use a short, shallow breath in labor. Short breaths that engage only your chest and not your abdomen are helpful in easing the baby through without tearing the perineum (the skin between your vagina and anal opening). Talk with your doctor or midwife about this part of the delivery and ask them to assist you with panting or any other methods to assure maximum stretchability of the vagina at delivery.

Crowning is usually a short part of the labor, accounting for no more than the last ten or fifteen minutes.

Massaging the Perineum Before Labor

Massaging your perineum fifteen to twenty minutes each day in the last month before delivery may help increase the blood supply to this area, making it more flexible during delivery. Gentle massaging all the way around the vagina in a circular manner with the fingertips can be done by yourself or by your partner. Some women enjoy using a light massage oil or cream to improve tissue tone. The goal is to maximize the natural capacity of your vagina to stretch easily around your baby's head. It is also an exercise that familiarizes you with your femininity and relaxes cultural taboos against women enjoying and knowing their own bodies. Exploring your vaginal area is an important part of knowing yourself and becoming comfortable with the labor and birth process.

Third Stage: The Placenta

The final stage of labor occurs after your baby is born. This is the last contraction and one you can look forward to because it does not hurt. It is simply the final contraction of labor as the placenta separates and slides out easily.

This last contraction usually occurs within twenty minutes after delivery. Your uterus will continue to contract down to its prepregnant size in the hours and days following birth. Your doctor or midwife will massage your womb to check its hardness and you will feel some cramping as the uterus shrinks.

You may want to save the placenta to look at later or freeze it until you can plant it under a tree. If so, be sure to ask your labor attendants to save it for you.

Now that you are familiar with the stages of labor it is time to consider your family relationships in your plans for giving birth.

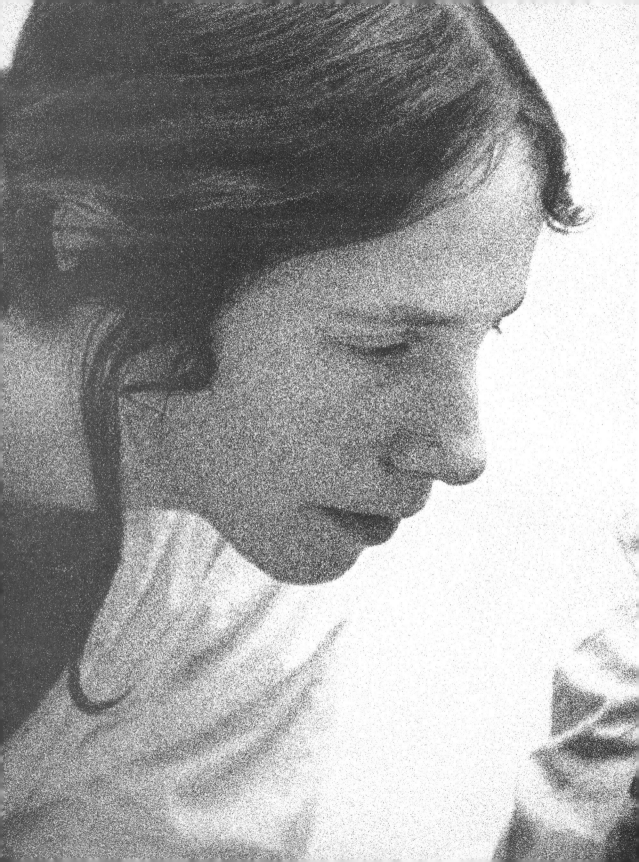

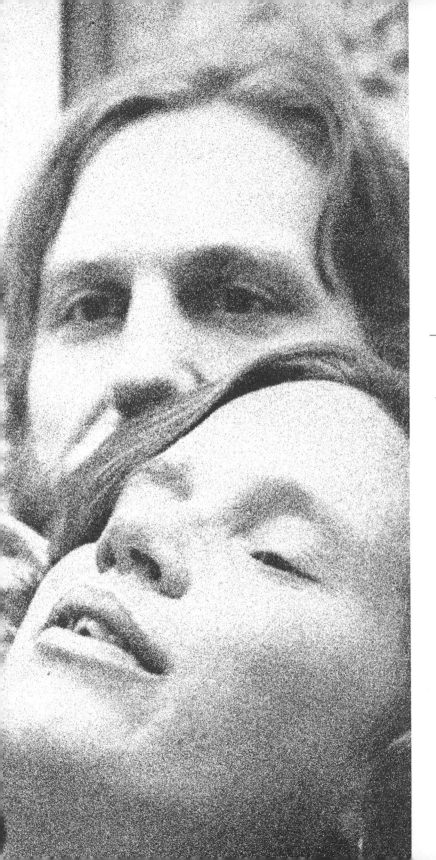

6

Coping
with Labor
Together

*But let there be spaces
in your togetherness,
and let the winds
of heaven
dance
between you*
KAHLIL GIBRAN
The Prophet

LABOR IS A MICROCOSM of life. It brings pain and pleasure, sadness and joy. Labor will put you in touch with both your strength and your dependency and offer you an opportunity to learn more about yourself. Sometimes we are happy with ourselves, other times we are not. Labor is not a time to judge ourselves but a period for reflecting on our movement through life at a given moment. It is not possible to control labor, it is only possible to follow the process and to meet whatever it may offer.

Labor is also teamwork. It is a mother and baby learning together how to push and how to be born, how to yield and separate from the union of pregnancy. You are not in control nor are you out of control during labor. The best way to approach labor is with an attitude of learning rather than controlling. This book presents an approach based on nature's cooperative energy, focusing on the harmony of mind and body—not mind over labor. An experientially based method of childbirth allows you to stay close to your body, using internal indicators of change instead of the clock. This allows you and your partner to enjoy early labor, which can be a lovely and even romantic time.

As contractions come and go, you can relax and sink into what I call laborland. Although somewhat painful at their peak, early labor contractions can border on pleasure and excitement. If you remain relaxed and breathing and if you are well-prepared, early labor can approach a quality of bliss. Cares can drift away as you sink into the deep pleasure of being with your partner—heart and mind.

Your Partner's Role during Labor

Witnessing the woman he loves in the middle of intense and painful contractions may be a very new experience for your partner. It is a natural response to want to take the pain away, to make it better for those we love and cherish. Sometimes a partner will feel afraid or guilty that he cannot share the pain. You must address these feelings before labor, so that they do not inhibit your coping abilities or distract your energy.

Reading this chapter together can help you develop a pattern for relating during labor that does not inhibit your ability to cope with pain. It helps to establish realistic expectations of each other and to open channels for communicating your needs. You need to be supported and encouraged to deal with contractions during active labor and not protected from normal pain.

You will find your energy diverted if your partner is so uncomfortable with your expressions of pain that instead of encouraging you, he only wants to stop your pain. This often happens when a partner takes on too much responsibility for his part in the process. First-time fathers often feel helpless when they expect more of themselves than is possible. A husband's job is to comfort and encourage, not to make the pain go away. It is a mistake for either of you to expect that your partner knows any more about labor than you do, or that he can lessen your pain or protect you from all intrusions—medical or otherwise. Neither of you should expect this to be his role.

If you have concerns about medical interventions, consider involving a trained labor or childbirth assistant. It is always a good idea to have available a knowledgeable person who can support you and your partner. Too often women express regret that their husbands did not know enough to comfort them during labor; some even end up angry at their partners. A husband may feel he failed when his wife's expectations for his role were not realistic. This common pitfall can be avoided by having a support person present who can tell you that what you are experiencing is normal and healthy. Taking time to read this chapter and to participate in the exercises in this book will give you a more realistic orientation.

It is also important to stop taking care of anyone else while you are in labor, including your partner. This is not a time when you can afford to inhibit your expression or the release of your pain. Do not play the role of hostess. Labor is a time when you owe all your attention and loving concern to yourself.

You and your partner are learning about the process of labor together. By sharing your fears and expectations, you can eliminate any false beliefs about comfort or protection that either of you may have. This can clear the way for loving support that is possible and realistic. True intimacy can make a difference in the quality of your journey into the unknown. The foundations for intimacy are honesty and sharing. Whatever your labor brings, it can be a shared experience that deepens your relationship rather than an isolating experience that alienates you from each other. How you travel through labor together can make all the difference as you begin your new family.

Building Trust and Open Communication

Set aside a special time to talk with your partner about the coming birth. What are his expectations, fears, and hopes? Tell him your own feelings, sharing with him what you are reading in this book.

Ask him to share his thoughts and feelings about seeing you in pain. How do you envision his support? Share this with him. How are your feelings, thoughts, and expectations similar? How do they differ?

Explore your different roles in labor. From what he knows of you, how does your partner expect you to cope? Does he have any fears or concerns about this? What do you expect of him? How does he feel about your expectations, fears, or desires? Does he feel he can give you what you expect to need from him in labor? If not, why not? Is what you are asking for realistic? Do you need an additional support person to help?

Discuss and explore these questions thoroughly. Adjust your plans accordingly. Simply listening to your partner's concerns can bring you closer, even if your ideal expectations of one another are not met. It is better to be real and honest with one another than to create false hopes that leave you both unprepared, hurt, and angry.

If this is a second or subsequent childbirth, take turns sharing your memory of the past childbirth experience(s). How did you feel about your partner during previous labor? How did he feel about you? About himself? Are there any feelings left over that need to be discussed? Understood? Forgiven? Appreciated? Anything you would like to do similarly or differently from before? For example, if your partner felt overwhelmed during a prior labor and was unable to offer you as much support as you needed, you may want to include plans for a childbirth assistant to support both of you next time.

Remember that no one can meet a partner's needs perfectly at all times. True intimacy is built on open communication with one another. The ability to ask and to hear is essential to building a foundation of trust together. We all have to be able to accept no as well as yes in answer to our needs. Intimacy requires that you be able to ask for your needs directly and that the other person be able to respond honestly.

A no does not mean your partner doesn't love you. It may simply mean he or she has human limits. What is important is the ability to communicate without blame and to find ways to share the experience in a positive way. By doing so, you will be creating a history of successes rather than failures.

Write down anything you learned from this exercise about yourself, your partner, and your communication skills. Are you able to express your needs? Are you able to accept responses you don't like? Can you be honest with each other about your limitations as well as your needs? Are you able to work together toward understanding each other, honoring limits, and finding ways to support one another? Include any new understanding of your partner that will help you in planning for the childbirth.

_____

_____

_____

_____

_____

_____

_____

_____

_____

_____

Other Children at the Birth

Siblings can benefit from being present at the birth of a baby if they are prepared for the process, and if quality care is provided during the labor so that your child's questions or needs are answered. General preparation for what to expect at the birth will contribute to your child's security and ability to bond with his or her sibling-to-be.

The first feelings to address are your own. As a mother you must feel comfortable with your child's presence at your labor. It is important that you not be distracted with worry about one child while you are laboring with another. If you feel a need to take care of the child while you are dealing with contractions, you will find it difficult to focus on your labor.

If you both feel comfortable with your child's presence, the next concern is that the child be prepared for birth through pictures, stories, and talking about the process. Special classes for siblings are available in some cities and can be particularly valuable for family bonding, whether or not the child actually attends the delivery.

Children need to be able to understand words in order to take preparation classes. Three years is the usual minimum age for a child attending a birth, but there is no evidence that younger children do not benefit. Some experts believe it potentially positive for children of any age to attend the birth of a sibling. However, it is also true that a negative experience can result if the child is improperly prepared or neglected during the event. A study by the Institute for Childbirth and Family Research in Madison, Wisconsin has identified the following guidelines for the presence of children at a birth. They can be applied to young children and teenagers alike. It is important that:

• The child is adequately prepared.

• The child wants to be present (for children who are old enough to express a desire).

• The child is cared for by an adult whose prime responsibility is to the child during the entire labor, and who enjoys a positive relationship with the child. The definition of "cared for" must match the child's needs. The needs of a teenager are different from those of a two year old, but both children need primary attention at this time.

• The child knows that he or she can have a change of heart at any time during labor or delivery and leave.

• The mother is comfortable with the child's presence during labor.

- The child is encouraged to interact with the baby in an appropriate manner soon after birth.

Each child is different, and there is no formula for family bonding. Talk with each other and research the resources in your area to decide whether having your child present for part or all of the birth is right for you and your family. Whether your child is present or not, it is important to include siblings in the preparations for the new baby. Choosing a name, helping to set up the basinette or nursery, or helping to pick out toys encourages sibling bonding. Talk together about ways you can prepare your child.

In the following spaces, write activities that you want to do with your older child(ren) that will contribute to healthy sibling attachment. Write your plans for caring for your child during labor.

Addressing Sibling Bonding before Delivery

1. How will you help your child prepare?

_____

_____

_____

_____

2. How will you include your child(ren) in the process of making room for a new baby?

_____

_____

_____

_____

_____

3. Who will be responsible for your child(ren) during labor?

_____

_____

Arrangements to have your child(ren) well cared for and prepared for birth will help you to relax during the last month of pregnancy. It will also allow you to turn your attention to your own preparation for labor, including dealing with the normal pain of childbirth.

Healthy Pain   The pain you will experience during labor is a healthy pain, not like the pain resulting from injury. It would be wonderful if English had more words for pain so that there would be a specific word for the kind that is productive and healthy. We can, however, teach ourselves a unique response to the pain of labor.

Labor pain is a natural and productive part of childbirth. It comes only intermittently and predictably. Contractions arise slowly, like ocean waves that you can hear coming from a distance. The release as the wave crashes and splashes to shore is inevitable. Then you and your baby can rest.

Fear can wash away as you understand the pain to be a natural part of a process. It is entirely manageable if you approach it realistically. A partner's role is simply to remind you that your cervix is dilating to a full ten centimeters. Since this does not happen at any other time, there will be a breakdown of tissue as it stretches and opens. It is natural for this to hurt. But the process is gradual; there are rests in between; and you can breathe through each contraction until it ebbs, as it inevitably will. Your partner should remind you that the pain is only an indication that your cervix is opening and the baby's head is coming down: It is a healthy sign that your baby is making headway through the cervix, through your vagina, and into your arms. It is a good and healthy pain that you can breathe through.

If your partner or childbirth assistant adopts this kind of comforting and encouraging attitude, you will find yourself able to deal with the contractions. You can also feel comforted and appreciated for the work you are doing.

The Baby's Journey   Keep in mind that during normal childbirth your baby does not feel pain. Although they are closely related, being born is a different process than giving birth. The baby does not have the pain of cervical dilation.

The baby's sensation is one of healthy stimulation—stress but not distress. Your baby is massaged by your uterine contractions, and you may think of your contractions as hugging your baby, as he or she moves through labor. Your contractions serve as a firm resistance for your baby to push off from as she or he presses into your cervix. Your baby has the ability to respond to the pressure of the contraction with a pushing reflex of its own. In this case, your baby presses with his or her feet against the force of the contraction, pushing its head down on the cervix. You can think of it as a child learning to swim, first crouching with feet on the wall of the pool, then pushing forcefully toward the center of the pool. In this way you and your baby work together during labor.

Your baby's head molds easily, fitting through the cervix as it opens. You might imagine how pleasant it can feel to have hands cupped around your head, as often happens during a massage. It feels good to have a certain amount of pressure on your head as the person's hands open and slide around the crown of your head, down over your ears, massaging your neck. And so it is for your baby.

Labor is naturally designed to stimulate your baby in preparation for breathing. As the baby comes down the birth canal, mucus is massaged out of the lungs so they will be ready to take in air at birth. The baby's circulatory system is stimulated by the friction of moving through the vagina, much as you stimulate warmth by rubbing your hands together on a cold day. This provides your baby with a fresh supply of blood, thus warming the skin, as it is born into a much cooler environment than it has known. Like many women, you may feel protective of your baby during labor. It can be comforting to visualize the normal labor process as a stimulating massage for your baby.

Having addressed concerns you may have had about your baby's experience during labor, you now continue preparing for labor. In the next chapter you will identify your natural coping style and build on this for an effective labor. You will also add new coping strategies to your current repertoire.

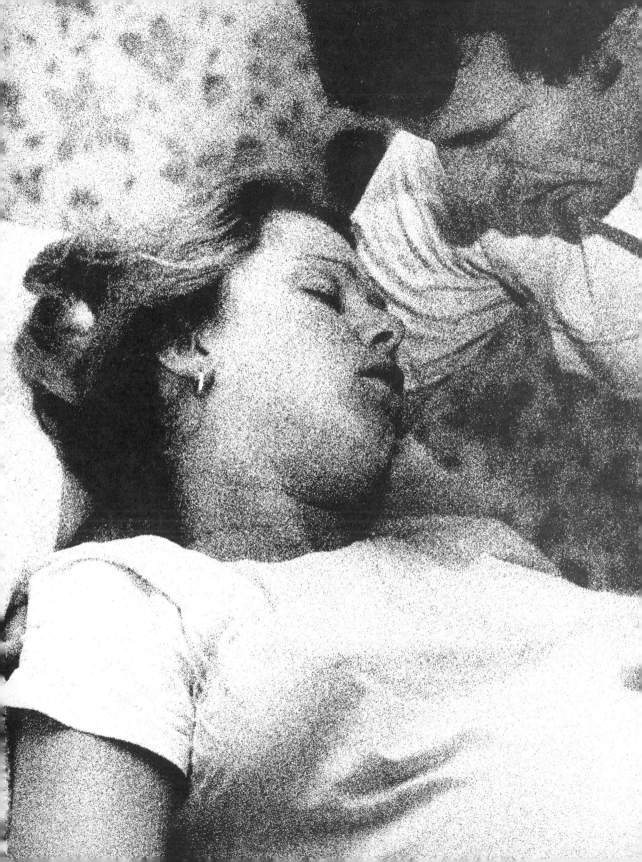

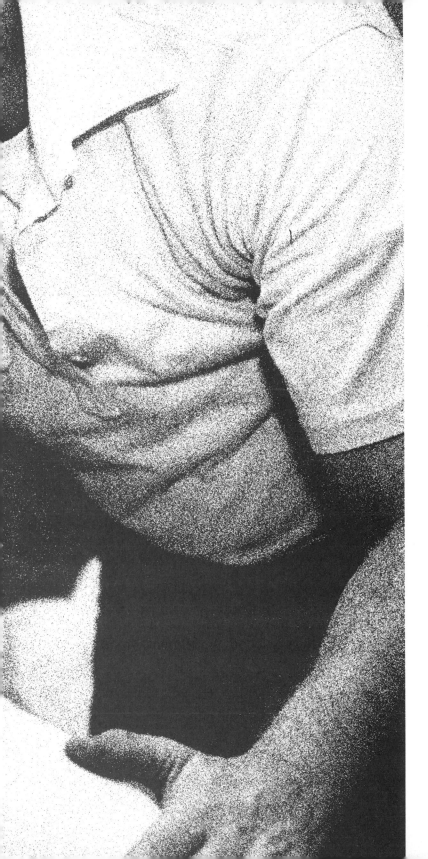

7

Coping with the Pain of Labor

I felt the pain travel through me and make way for the baby coming down. . . . I knew the pain was natural so I knew it was helping me . . . like a friend. I can honestly say there was no fear.

GABRIELLA
after her second labor

In our society we have not accepted pain as either a teacher or a friend, to learn from and grow with. Instead we are encouraged to take aspirin, sleeping pills, or tranquillizers—to flee from any possible hurt or discomfort. Although some pain control is helpful, there is also much lost when the coping style is one of automatic avoidance.

This pattern of coping by avoiding may be at the root of many addictions. These patterns of denial and avoidance have received much attention in the media. It is now widely acknowledged that our society has lost its coping skills. We have forgotten how to help each other tolerate pain that is natural, useful, and sometimes unavoidable.

When drugs for managing pain are necessary during labor, some of the rewards of natural birth are lost. When such drugs are needed, no woman's request should be refused. We often, however, fail women before they even begin labor by not realistically preparing them to cope.

Whether our expectations match reality has enormous impact on emotions. More important, the difference between reality and expectations affects our physiology. Depending on our emotions, the limbic system of our brains determines how much of a particular hormone is to be produced or released into the bloodstream.

Emotions and Labor The limbic system is often described as the emotional center of the brain because it sends messages to the body based on emotional arousal. Hormones, neurochemicals, and other substances are released according to an individual's perceptions of the world.

The limbic system responds to the perception of danger. Later, perhaps, the person observes that the danger was only an illusion, a shadow instead of a pursuer. The body, however, responds to the first impression of impending danger and only later to the reality of safety. Physiological chemistry returns to normal when the person resolves the emotional panic.

During labor, the hormone oxytocin is released by the pituitary gland. In addition, prostaglandins are circulated throughout the bloodstream, helping to soften the cervix as the oxytocin causes the uterus to contract. The amounts of oxytocin released and the secretion of hormones that control prostaglandins during labor are determined by the hypothalamus, which is affected by the limbic system. The brain regulates labor in response to many messages, including the woman's emotional state. Fear and anxiety during labor have been found to decrease the flow of oxytocin. In this way, emotional factors can influence your labor.

Women having first babies experience a higher incidence of labor dysfunction than do women who already know what to expect in labor, as well as motherhood. When women are able to match their expectations more closely with reality, they are better prepared for childbirth. The discrepancy between expectation and reality can produce high levels of fear and anxiety. Reducing this discrepency is one key to increasing your likelihood for normal delivery.

Expectation and Pain

The hippocampus, a part of the brain, has been found to mediate between the expectation of an experience and its actuality. As long as differences between what one expects and what is actually experienced remain minor, there is a stabilizing balance in hormonal and other brain-regulated activity. The limbic system has a tension relaxation dimension that becomes unbalanced, however, when what is expected deviates greatly from what is experienced.

The following exercises will guide you through realistic preparations that can help you master the fears that accompany childbirth. The visualization audiotape that you will create for yourself as you read chapter 8 will also serve to reach your emotional, or limbic, level of awareness. You will be able to add personal history and concerns to your birth visualization, thereby rendering it soothing and pertinent to your situation. In this way, you will prepare yourself emotionally for childbirth.

Separating Pain from Fear

During your final month of pregnancy you may view a variety of videos and films on childbirth. Using your resources (childbirth educator, birth center, obstetrician, midwife), locate a film or videotape that presents a realistic account of labor. It should document the mother's experience of pain and how she coped during contractions. You should be able to see and hear her pain, so that you can face your own emotional reaction prior to your childbirth, working through your anxieties ahead of time.

The film you choose should also depict a completely normal delivery so that you connect the normal pain of labor with birth. Viewing complications of birth at this time will distract you from dealing with normal pain, which is the point of this exercise. Complications can be addressed better after you have first dealt with the normal fears and anxieties.

This exercise has three components. The first is viewing a childbirth film with your partner and then sharing the feelings that the film brings up, particularly about your expectations of pain. For the second part of the exercise view it together again, a week or more later, after having worked through the feelings that surfaced during the first viewing.

The third part is done as you view the film both times, during which you identify with normal healthy labor, including the pain. In this part of the exercise you learn by association. Your intuitive mind absorbs information through identification, which is one way we prepare for new experience. Once birth was institutionalized, identification was not readily available as a means of learning about birth; films provide a good alternative.

Part One
When you have decided on a particular film, schedule a time to view it with your partner or a friend who will be with you during labor. Allot at least forty-five minutes afterward to share your feelings. The following questions and guidelines can facilitate your discussion.

1. Do you expect there will be pain during labor? Guideline: Be aware that not expecting it is unrealistic and should be seen as unproductive denial or wishful thinking by either partner. Work through any denial and deal with your fear if labor were to be painful.

2. Were you afraid during the viewing? What caused your fear? Guideline: Recognize that your fear as an observer is natural, but that the woman herself may not have been afraid. Pain is not fear. If you see a woman labor and later she tells you she was not afraid, you learn intuitively that fear does not necessarily accompany pain. This has been my own experience and that of many women I have worked with over the years. Work to separate your fear from the healthy pain of labor. Dealing with pain when it is part of a normal process is merely a matter of coping with it.

3. How did you see the woman on the film manage the pain during contractions? Guideline: Include any ways that you might imagine yourself or your partner dealing with contractions. Remind yourself that you can do it, as have women throughout history.

4. How do you think you will cope with pain during labor? What might you need from your partner or from others? Guideline: Keep in mind that if neither of you has gone through or been present at a labor before, you may both need support. Who will be there for your partner? It is not realistic for either of you to expect that your partner will be able to do or be everything for you, from easing the pain to dealing with medical interventions and decisions. Your partner can comfort you and support you, but neither of you should confuse this with taking away the physical pain of labor.

5. What can you expect from your partner during labor? Guideline: Your partner may support you best by reminding you that the contraction will ebb soon, and that the force of the contraction is helping your baby come down the birth passage. This prevents him from feeling helpless and wanting the labor to stop, and it keeps you from losing perspective. Your partner's job is to remind you that the pain is helping to open the cervix, and that it means that the baby is on its way.

6. How did you feel when the woman shown in the film was finally holding her baby in her arms? Guideline: Keep in mind that this is where you are heading. Imagine what your partner will look like holding your newborn. Close your eyes and see these pictures.

Part Two
View the film again, approximately one week later. This
will give you time to process what you discovered; you will
find your second viewing somewhat different. Share your
reactions again, noting the changes you sense as you identify your feelings and your fear begins to dissolve. Discuss
your feelings with each other until your anxiety lessens and
your confidence in yourself increases.

Part Three
As you view the film, identify with the woman going
through a totally normal and painful experience. You can
be assured that you too can deal with the normal and
healthy pain of labor. Repeat this message to yourself as
you watch. Pay attention, however, to your own feelings as
they come up. Note any fears or anxiety, pleasure or excitement as you hear and see her work to deliver her baby.

Be certain that the film shows a normal labor and birth,
as well as graphically illustrates her pain and hard work.
By identifying with her, you will already be adjusting to
pain and emotionally linking it with normality. Confronting this experience provides you with an opportunity to
desensitize yourself emotionally to pain during labor.
When you do so, fear begins to fade and you begin to
expect pain without fear. This is the key.

Your Natural
Coping Style
You will need to improve your ability to cope with the
contractions of active labor. To meet these stronger contractions more easily, you need to understand your own
style of taking in new information.

People have three major channels for receiving information. Based in the three sensory cortices of the brain,
they are: auditory, visual, and kinesthetic. From the time
of birth, we each develop unique patterns for processing
and organizing information. Psychologists John Grinder
and Richard Bandler, in their two volumes of *The Structure
of Magic*, analyzed patterns by which people process experience. They describe these models as representational
systems, and they believe that people will lead with one
and favor one, or possibly two, cortices when they incorporate new information.

Some people process information using the internal, or secondary, visual cortex, which is used in dreaming and visualization. For them, seeing is believing. Others rely on the secondary auditory cortex and repeat phrases in order to comprehend a concept. People who utilize their secondary auditory cortex in this way will be likely to use such auditory metaphors as 'It rings true.' Still others use the internal kinesthetic cortex as their primary way to process new information. These people may need a hunch—or a gut feeling—in order to understand.

It is also possible, even desirable, to develop all three cortices for information processing. The ability to do so yields greater creativity and lends a richness to our everyday experience. The cortex we use for initial processing, however, will be the system we lead with and therefore our predominant style for integrating new information in a managcable manner.

When we can identify our primary channel for receiving information, we can enhance our natural coping style for dealing with pain in labor. Some women suppress their natural style because they have been taught relaxation and breathing techniques that do not take into account their unique way of processing the labor experience.

Women have many different ways of dealing with pain during labor. When left to uninhibited expression, a large percentage will moan or make some use of sound during labor. These women use an auditory means of expression for dealing with their pain. Other women may squeeze a pillow or a friend's hand or even want to move around as a way of meeting the contractions. These women are kinesthetic in their coping style. Still others prefer to use internal or externalized visual images for traveling through contractions. These women primarily use a visual means of coping with pain.

Some methods of childbirth preparation inhibit vocalization or movement because these expressions do not fit the concepts of what relaxation is supposed to look or sound like. Methods that discourage sound and squeezing in favor of visual relaxation techniques that render a woman quiet and still often inhibit her natural or predominant coping style. Because labor is so intense most women need to work through a contraction with auditory or kinesthetic techniques in addition to visual methods.

The following exercises will help you to understand and identify your own natural coping style. They will also increase your ability to develop your other sensory pathways for dealing with pain during contractions.

Identifying Your Primary System

Lie down comfortably, perhaps on your side with a pillow between your legs to accommodate the space between your hips, which is widening now that you are very pregnant. This exercise is best done when you are approximately seven months pregnant. At this time you are eager to prepare for birth, and learning comes quickly.

Arrange for your partner or a friend to pinch you on the fleshy part of your leg behind your knee. You will feel pain and you will have to accommodate it in some way. Instruct your partner to gradually, over the course of sixty seconds, increase the pressure of the pinch until he or she is pinching you very hard. The pinch simulates a contraction in that it causes you to do something, either internally or externally, to adjust to it. If it does not challenge you, then your partner is being too gentle. You should feel a need to respond in some way to allow the pain to be present and then pass.

Give yourself sixty seconds to rest and relax before the next simulated contraction. Relaxing between contractions is a very important part of the exercise.

Partner's instructions. **Pinch under the knee, building from a gentle squeeze to a hard pinch in thirty seconds. Talk her through the simulated contraction, telling her that you are about to begin to squeeze before you do, then telling her when it is peaking and when it is beginning to fade. When you reach the maximum pinch at thirty seconds, hold the pressure for approximately ten seconds, telling her it has peaked, then gradually loosen your hold, diminishing the squeeze, while telling her it is fading. The gradual fading should take twenty seconds. You should observe your partner exerting some effort to deal with the pain when it is peaking.**

How did you respond to the pain? Did you hold your breath? Did you breathe harder, listening to your breath and your partner's voice? (auditory) Did you speak to your-self internally? (auditory) Did you tighten your hands into a fist? (kinesthetic) Did you use movement of any kind, such as hitting your hand on the couch? (kinesthetic) Did you want a cold or a hot compress? (kinesthetic) Did you use images to help you? Perhaps nature scenes? (visual) Or sounds, such as rushing water? (auditory) Or faces of those you love? (visual) . . . If necessary, do the exercise again paying particular attention to your responses. If you found that you instinctively held your breath, do the exercise again, being certain to continue your breathing while observing what other ways you respond.

You already may have identified whether your instinctive response is auditory, visual, or kinesthetic. The following exercises will help you to clarify which modalities will work best for you during labor. I encourage you to try all three, as well as combinations of auditory-kinesthetic, and auditory-visual-kinesthetic to see what works best for you.

If there are any medical contraindications to this exercise, such as varicose veins, consult your doctor.

Auditory Coping

The only negative way of coping is holding your breath. Sometimes you won't notice you are doing so because it is instinctive, especially if you have been taught to hold in your feelings and not express yourself. It is important to continue breathing through contractions. One way for your partner to know for sure you are breathing is if he can hear it.

Women who stifle their breathing usually have a conditioned response to hide pain or do not want to cause distress to others. Remember that this is your labor. Do what works for you and let others take care of themselves. If your tendency is to hold back, work toward expression and release. By doing so, you will be getting ready for labor.

Do the simulated contraction again, this time purposely giving some sound to your breath. Hissing is good because it engages the diaphragm, even though during labor you would use a moan instead of hissing, because the internal pressure of the contraction would be present. A low humm or hiss is best for this exercise.

When the pinch begins to peak, use the sound of your

breathing to carry you through it. Increase the hiss to a very loud sound. Put all the pain into the sound of your breath, making it louder the more pain you feel. Let the sound diminish as the pain ebbs and you no longer need the sound to help you.

Kinesthetic Coping

Some women confront pain with movement, perhaps squeezing a pillow or even their partner's hand. As long as you are breathing, movement is a useful technique for traveling through contractions. When women hold their breath, however, they are also squeezing inside.

It is entirely possible to squeeze or tighten your fist without tensing the internal organs. Your muscles and voluntary nervous system do not necessarily affect your uterus. If you are furrowing your brow, say, unfurrowing it will not be better for labor. In fact it is unrealistic for women to expect they will totally relax all muscles during a contraction. Women who cope kinesthetically usually need to express their pain physically. By squeezing a pillow with your hand, you can express this tension externally, thereby lessening the likelihood of inner tension. As long as you continue to breathe, your physical expression will help you through the contraction.

Repeat the simulated contraction with your partner, this time using the squeezing technique to express and release pain at the peak of the contraction. You may also want to use both auditory and kinesthetic responses, particularly if you are inclined to hold your breath.

Visual Coping

When using visual imagery for coping with contractions, it is important that the image change or transform in some way to match the changing intensity of the simulated contraction. If you are using the image of a flower opening, say, you should visualize the flower opening larger, or its color deepening, as the contraction peaks. This allows the secondary visual cortex to accommodate the increased sensation of the simulated contraction.

Repeat the simulated contraction, this time using an internal image that changes as the contraction peaks. Be sure you are breathing throughout the exercise.

None of these techniques will work if you hold your breath. That is why it is often a good idea to incorporate hearing the sound of your breath during contractions no matter what other modalities you use or favor.

Try the exercise again. This time listen to the sound of your breathing, imagine your baby's head coming down as your cervix opens, and hold tight to your partner's hand. This allows you to experience all three coping strategies. Of these, which comes most naturally to you? Which helps most with the pain? Can you use each of them or all three together? These coping strategies will be helpful when you have entered active labor. Use these techniques when you need something more than deep breathing during either the first or second stage of labor.

By doing the above exercises just one time thoroughly, you have trained your body to adjust and adapt by using pain to help you through labor. Your body will automatically respond to what works for you in these hands-on, body-centered exercises.

Experience is almost always the best teacher. These exercises are part of your experiential preparation; what you learn becomes instinctual. The next time you need to cope with pain—in any form—this repertoire of responses will spring to the forefront of your consciousness. Many women use the coping strategies learned in childbirth to achieve a calm through later periods of stress, whether physical or emotional. The preparation you are doing for childbirth will continue to benefit you throughout life.

Relaxation and Release

Remember to relax between contractions. During a contraction, encourage yourself to meet its peak with the strategies that work for you. Do not expect yourself to be totally relaxed during the height of a contraction; use your best coping strategies to release pain. You will find yourself adjusting to your own inner tempo. Welcome the deep rest that is possible between contractions. It is within these peaceful valleys that you can replenish yourself. Some women even report falling asleep between contractions.

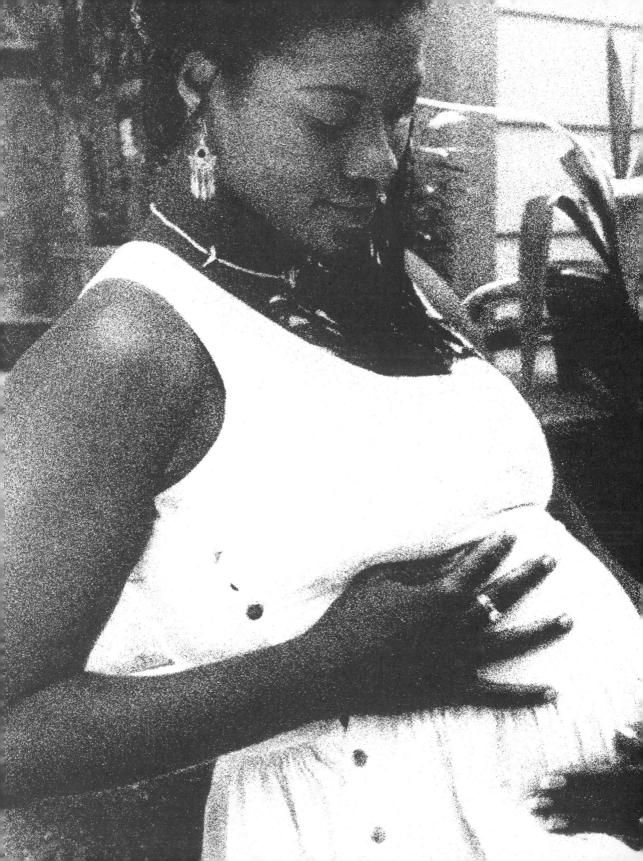

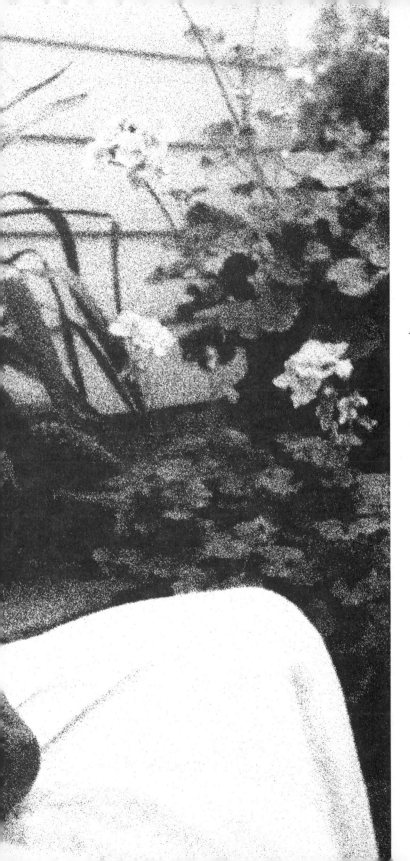

8

Relaxation and Visualization for Childbirth

*Her vagina . . . stretched wide open
as the top of your head slid out.
Then the rest of your head
slipped out and it turned,
and a shoulder slid out
and then the other . . .
You could open your eyes and
see your mother . . .*

SHEILA KITZINGER
Being Born

READ THE FOLLOWING EXERCISE and write in the space provided the suggestions that are appropriate to your situation. You may want to refer to your birth-preparation inventory in chapter 1 to review the issues associated with your childbirth. You can then read the relaxation and birth visualization into a tape recorder for replay or have another person read it to you. This way you can relax and absorb the suggestions given.

Once you have created the tape, set aside an hour to relax and listen to it. Wear loose, comfortable clothing and remove glasses or hard contact lenses before beginning. Feel free to change your position as you fall deeper into a relaxed state. Your body will guide you into a more comfortable position as you listen. Adjusting your position can release tension as you take in the suggestions.

Do not begin using the relaxation-visualization tape until you are in your last month of pregnancy. By then you will be ready to absorb the suggestions in the birth visualization and less likely to hold yourself back from the experience. If you have a tendency toward premature labor or should earliest labor have begun without your knowledge, waiting will ensure that you will not intensify your body's response to contractions. Although visualization does not precipitate labor, it can encourage the process once it begins. Consult your doctor or midwife if you have concerns about using the tape too early.

Visualization can also help calm your mind and resolve fears. When labor begins you will be able to call upon the metaphors used in your visualization to help you.

Instructions for the Visualizations

The visualization transcripts are best read in a soft, steady voice with special emphasis where needed. If a word is italicized, it should be stressed. Where indicated, the italicized word should convey the feeling of the word; for example, "heavy" should be spoken in a way that suggests heaviness. This helps the pregnant woman absorb the suggestions deeply. The more you can evoke the sensation of the word, the greater the effectiveness of visualization. Dots (. . .) indicate where the reader should pause to give the woman time to absorb the suggestion.

You will occasionally be reading phrases rather than whole sentences. Do not be surprised by sequences that are ungrammatical. The brain's right hemisphere, the part that registers feelings and spatial relationships, absorbs suggestions best when they are phrased with tonality, texture, and pauses. Whoever is making the recording should read the passages through once before taping. Be aware that suggestions travel deeper into your subconscious as they are repeated. Hearing phrases again and again while in a relaxed state is an excellent technique for reaching the inner mind. Remember that you are addressing the emotional hemisphere of the brain, so keep the flow of your voice consistent and steady. Read the exercise as you would read poetry aloud. The occasional headlines, such as "Relaxation Preparation," are not to be said aloud. They are merely signals for the reader.

When you are creating your own suggestions be sure that you couch them in metaphors that first state the problem, then resolve it. One example is a rough, graveled road (which represents a difficult first birth) changing to a smoother, paved road. Refer to the audio and visual tapes on body-centered hypnosis listed at the back of this book for examples of birth visualizations. Use your imagination and enjoy yourself. Begin . . .

Relaxation Preparation

Just as you have adapted and adjusted to the pregnancy, your body continues to adjust and adapt in order to bring your baby out. In fact, you can, _____, think of labor as a process of adjustment, whereby your cervix stretches around your baby's head as he or she comes down your vagina and your pelvic ligaments adjust in response to the hormone relaxin, which increases in your bloodstream near the end of the pregnancy. It will be helpful to give yourself the suggestion that you are just beginning to follow your baby now, through the changes necessary to give birth. Slowly your hormones shift and rearrange during the last month of pregnancy and you can, _____, feel your baby's head heavy, down on your cervix.

To personalize. **In the above sequence and throughout the tape, insert your first name into the blanks and, if you wish, in other places. The inner mind pays special attention when your name is spoken.**

Begin by listening to your breath now. Coming in, going out. Take yourself just a little bit deeper down into your breathing. As you breathe in you take in what you need for yourself, _____. The oxygen absorbed into the deep cellular structure of each and every organ. Without your even needing to direct it or think about it. As you breathe out you let go of carbon dioxide, toxins. Tension can just begin to flow out of you. A little more and a little more with each breath out.

And now you can, if you like, _____, take that just a bit *deeper* now. Breathing in all that you need for yourself. Oxygen, flowing easily, nourishing your body now. Exhaling, breathing out what's not needed, carbon dioxide, tension, worries can just begin to let go. You just don't need them right now. You can put aside the tension you don't need as you relax, as you listen to this tape now. An island of time floating, carries you, like a hammock supporting you, _____, between two strong trees. And you don't need to go anywhere or do anything but just *be*. Supported by the hammock, releasing into the strong support of the two trees now.

So that with your next breath, you can become aware of the breath traveling from your left shoulder, _____, right down through into the elbow and even deeper down through to the wrist and hand, right out the fingertips. So that your left arm now can just begin to let go, to relax a little more, and a little more on the inside without your even needing to think about it now. Your baby's arm also relaxes, baby's arms relaxing inside the waters, _____, inside your womb, now.

There was a time when you were inside your own mother's womb. Inside the waters. And inside the waters, _____, you could hear the beating of your mother's heart. You could hear those sounds through the waters, just as your baby can hear the sound of your heartbeat. And even as you relax the right shoulder in the same way, just beginning to breathe out any tension from your right shoulder right down through to the elbow and even deeper down through to the wrist and hand, right out through the fingertips. So that both arms, _____, like your baby's arms, begin to let go, to relax a little more, and a little more with each breath out. As your baby grows on the inside, as your baby knows how to grow without your even needing to think about it, on the inside, you can take yourself right down into the hips, which have actually spread outward in space. Your hips have spread outward to make a cradling space, cradling your baby deep. Deep, deep inside your pelvis, even deeper than the month before, deeper than the month before that.

So that with your next breath, _____, just continue to breathe out any tension not needed from your right hip, right down through your thigh, to your knee. And with your next breath even deeper down through to your ankle, your foot and right out your toes. So that your right leg can just begin to let go, relax.

Now bring your focus to your left hip in the same way, just beginning to breathe out any tension from the left hip, _____, right down through your thigh to your knee. And even deeper down through your ankle and foot and right out your toes. So that your left leg too can just begin to let go, a little more and a little more with each breath down and out.

With your next breath you can, _____, feel free to focus on your throat now. The throat is a very important part of the body, especially during childbirth. Related to your vagina. So that with your next breath you can just imagine what it might look like inside as your throat begins to loosen and relax a little more with each breath out and down. And as you breathe you can imagine the oxygen, follow it right into your lungs, becoming aware that as you breathe in your chest rises a bit . . . and as you breathe out it falls a bit . . . rises . . . and falls . . . So that as your chest expands you actually create more space inside . . . for your heart, your lungs . . . for every organ to adjust and find the healthiest position at any given moment in time.

So that with your next breath you can begin to travel to your stomach now. Your stomach is an incredibly adjustable and resilient organ. It knows how to move up and out of the way as the baby grows. Without you even needing to think about it, your stomach knows how to adjust, to yield to your baby on the inside. Just begin to breathe out any tension from your stomach now, so that it can become calm. Like a calm peaceful lake, in which you could skip a stone and watch the circles spread . . . outward and . . . outward . . . smoother and smoother now.

So that with your next breath you can, _____, travel down into your vagina now. As if you could breathe in through your throat and right out through your vagina. In through your throat and out through the vagina. Clearing the way for a very smooth, open passageway . . . for birth.

So that with your next breath, come to a place on the back of your neck. Just beginning to travel down your spine, letting your breath massage the inside of your backbone as you travel from the first vertebra, slipping and sliding smoothly down to the second, the third . . . all the way down to the middle of your back. Sinking slower and deeper down through your lower back, all the way down through your tailbone. You might even remember a time when you slid down a slide. The very first time, or the second time in your life . . . climbing up the ladder, step by step to the very top. Perhaps there was someone there to help you, _____, so that you were not afraid. And you were clinging very tightly to the slide, but with encouragement you *let go* . . . and right down the slide you came, so smooth and so fast. . . . And it was so much fun, that you went around again, learning how to let go at the top . . . all the way down to the bottom. It was so much fun!

To personalize. **Create your own suggestion for transforming past difficulty either in previous childbirth or with your own birth. Make a version of the slide metaphor that fits your circumstances and creates a positive possibility for your coming delivery. For example, if you had a difficult first birth, see the**

initial journey down the slide as difficult, but create a smoother glideway the second time down. Refer to your birth inventory for concerns about your own birth or previous childbirth that can be worked through in the slide metaphor. Your inner mind will respond to the message you give it, helping to relax you during labor.

_____

_____

_____

_____

_____

_____

_____

_____

    With your next breath you can, _____, return to that point on the back of your neck. This time just letting the relaxation spread . . . up your scalp . . . down your forehead, so that your eyebrows can drift . . . farther and farther apart. Letting the relaxation spread right down your face and jaw, right through to your throat again, breathing out any tension from your throat and traveling, following your breath as it travels down into your womb right now.

And as you breathe now your baby, _____, knows how to release, to adjust itself, to move on the inside. You might even feel your baby moving now. Sink down into your breathing, deepening your rest as if your breath, like the hammock, could support you, safely and surely support you as your body releases into the hammock now. Knowing that as you breathe in, all the oxygen needed travels right through the cord into your baby. As you breathe, follow the oxygen right _down_ into the placenta now. Your breath knows how to travel. The oxygen travels easily through the placenta, through the cord, _____, into your baby without your even needing to think about it. So that you can imagine what it actually looks like on the inside, _____, inside the womb now. You can give yourself the right to see what your baby might

Bonding with Your Baby in the Womb

look like. Little handprints, tiny footprints all its own. Like no other baby that has ever come before. Can look deep, *deep* into your baby's eyes. Say Hello. Giving yourself the right to, _____, *feel* the love that already exists between you even now. This baby is coming into your life now, making family. It's supposed to be coming to you, to _____, your partner, whatever the timing. The right time to be born.

To personalize. **Insert your partner's name in the previous blank. If your situation varies, such as single parenthood or an unmarried partnership, change the sentence accordingly, putting in names of people who your baby will know as family when he or she is born.**

Your body knows if you're growing a boy or a girl, knows how, _____, knows how to make that baby on the inside as it grows, beginning to grow into family now, another person in the family, already on the inside of your body now. You can *feel* the baby's knee and foot and hand press through the waters, through the bag of water inside your womb. The inside cells of your womb are actually touching your baby on the inside now. As if you could, _____, *touch* your baby, as if you could touch your baby's forehead with your lips, with a kiss. Without even needing to think about it now, baby knows how to settle deep, deep, deep into the pelvis, as the baby gets ready to be born. Your hips adjust, _____, adjust and adapt around the baby's head as it descends down, *down* just a little more, just a little more, with each hour closer and *closer* to the time when your baby will come right *down* on the inside of the cervix. At the right time, just as flowers bloom in spring, and rain *falls* to the earth. Without your even needing to think about it.

Now take yourself forward in time as if through a time tunnel to the birth day, _____, the day of your baby's birth. A day you will be celebrating next year, and the year after that, and the year after that. Perhaps it will be the day you are due, perhaps a few days later, _____, or maybe even _____, several days before.

To personalize. **Fill in the previous blanks with your due date and the dates for a day or two immediately before and after this date.**

As the birth day draws near, _____, your cervix is getting softer, like a pear ripens on a tree. And *heavier*, and the tree wants to let go of that pear but the pear is just waiting there, just right, just waiting for exactly the right time, getting *fuller*, getting *softer* as it ripens. You can feel that pear begin to *soften* like the cervix does a little more and a little more after thirty-six weeks even more at thirty-eight weeks, may begin to soften. And your baby is getting ready to dive right down, deeper and *deeper* down. Your body adjusts and adapts to follow, _____, follow, follow your baby.

Birth Visualization

Note to the reader. **Remember to use your voice to make the words in italics sound like what they feel like. "Softer" should sound soft and "heavier" should be said in such a way as to convey heaviness. In this way, the inner mind takes in the sensation of the visualized images, which greatly increases the effectiveness of these suggestions.**

And there will come a time, _____, when you can feel your baby's head coming right down on your cervix, at just the right time, like that pear knows when, knows when to fall *thud* right down to the ground. There will come a time, when the baby just begins to know when to be born. On the inside a kind of body knowledge getting ready, getting ready to dive right down through, right through the vagina, right through the tunnel way. Right through, _____, and into your arms! You can feel good to know your baby is getting ready, getting ready to be born, to dive down through the soft tissue of your vagina.

As the baby gets ready, sometimes at thirty-nine weeks or thirty-nine and a half weeks and sometimes at forty weeks, and I don't know exactly when for you, _____, you'll become due, and the baby will want to come out, want to be born into the world to see you now, making family, making a family, weaving and weaving the basket now, weaving the basket of family. The basket of family now, safely, safely, there.

To personalize. **Make your own suggestion for resolving feelings about a difficult birth now. You can use a metaphor that transforms a past birth into the experience you want to have with your next, such as a journey down a road that was rough and covered with gravel but now is paved with asphalt, offering a smoother and faster journey. Personalize your suggestion so that you can use a prior birth as a resource for your next one. Refer to your birth inventory to review past childbirth. Write the suggestion and metaphor in the space provided. Make it a part of your personal relaxation tape.**

_____

_____

_____

_____

_____

_____

_____

_____

_____

_____

_____

Contractions Are Like Ocean Waves

As the baby begins to dive down, _____, you feel contractions coming and going and going and coming, then another contraction is building, you can feel it building. Like waves coming safely to shore, they come and they go. Bringing the baby down. Contractions are hugging the baby and helping your baby clear the way, _____, clear the way through.

But then the contractions begin to build stronger and faster, stronger and faster, than the ones before. Just like the waves in the ocean know how to come to shore and wash clear and wash clean. You can *use* that energy, that energy of the waters, as you feel the contraction coming. It's as if the wave was building deep deep in the depths of the ocean, before anyone else knows that you know it's coming, *feel* your baby diving and diving and *diving* right down on the cervix. But then the wave comes to shore and you rest and your baby rests, in between each and every contraction. Gathering energy, resting deeply. In between each contraction, _____, you can sink down, sink down and rest deeply and completely. Plenty of time to rest in between contractions. Remember that.

And then you can feel the next contraction, _____, like a wave moving and *moving* the baby down and you begin to breathe and breathe and the baby's diving and *diving* right down, right down on the cervix now you can feel yourself breathe and breathe and the baby's diving and diving and opening and opening the cervix, can feel it open and *open*.

Reminder to reader. **The reader should alter the voice, again to convey the sensation of diving and opening as much as possible.**

But then the wave splashes to shore, _____, crashes and *splashes* safely to shore. You can feel that energy *deep* on the inside running deeper and deeper inside of your body now. As your baby rests in between each and every contraction, can feel your baby's head sink down a little more, and a little more, in between each and every contraction. The waves always come to shore, they always come to shore. You can remember that during labor, can remember that they always come to shore and you can, _____, rest deep inside. Gathering strength, energy as your baby rests, getting ready, getting ready, getting ready for the next contraction. But in between you can drift and shift and sift and dip down into the ocean as the wave curls backward and into the sea gathering, gathering what's needed on the inside so that with the next contraction you can feel refreshed and revitalized. . . .

But then you can feel the wave building and feel it surging, _____, deep on the inside, the wave begins to gather and gather and gather, can feel your baby begin to move right down on the cervix, and the cervix begins to open and open and *open* and the baby's diving and diving and *diving* right down on the cervix now. You can feel that wave building and building, _____, smooth and sure, can feel the wave building and building and the baby's diving and diving and diving *full* force safely down now, opening, opening the cervix and you're breathing and breathing right through the contraction. And you can feel the wave wash and wash and *wash* to the shore now, _____, wash into the shore now, crashes and, *splashes* free as your baby moves down, down deeper and deeper down, deeper and deeper down through the cervix. You can feel your cervix opening and opening a little more and a little more with each dip down of the contractions, _____, you can feel good, good in between, almost like a flower opening on the inside, opening a pink rose opening, opening in the rain. *Feel* the raindrop if you were that flower, *feel* the raindrop *slide* right down deep into the very inner, inner depths, inner depths of that rose that *wants* to open. The rose wants to open to the sky, _____, and your cervix opens to your baby now, to your baby on the inside. And the waters are calm now, calm and deep. And still . . . in between each and every contraction you rest and your baby rests. . . .

And contractions come and go, go and come. Like waves, they surge and dip on the inside, safely, safely coming to shore each time. And just as the rose opens, _____, in springtime, it's just a matter of time. A matter of time, until the rose is completely open to the sky. It knows how to open itself on the inside. It's inevitable . . . opening to your baby now. . . .

And then another contraction is building, and you can, _____, *feel* the wave safely surging and surging and *surging*, can feel your baby diving and diving and *diving* right down on your cervix as it opens, completely open and free right around your baby's head. And you breathe and breathe and your baby dives and dives right down and through the cervix. Opening completely now, until the wave splashes to shore, _____, and it always comes to shore each and every wave, always comes to shore, you can remember that during labor, _____, that each wave always comes to shore and you rest . . . always adjusting and adapting to the waves moving on the inside. You rest, and your baby rests always sinking down, letting time carry you. Time carries you, swiftly and deeply now, knows how to carry you down deep, deep down to the very bottom of the ocean where all the trace elements known and still unknown are on the very bottom of the ocean and in your baby's body, too. Every time you rest in between a contraction can feel as if you sink down to the replenishment available to you. The colors, the light coming through the ocean waters can carry you, _____, down into the deep deep colors of the coral and the fish, all the elements needed in the seaweed are there for you, exist on the very bottom of the ocean, there are even little sea animals generating lights all their own, different colored lights on the very bottom, schools of fish, each one with a mother, schools of fish born to their mothers on the very bottom of the ocean. And these fish *move*, _____, on the currents of the water and gather what's needed, gather what's needed from the sea. Like the waters inside your womb, _____, help you ... adjust, adapt, yield to the movement of the contractions during labor. . . .

And your baby, _____, begins to dive through the vagina getting very ready, very stimulated, very healthy, feels *good* to a baby to come right down through the vagina, right down through the tissue, the billowy, pillowy, willowy tissue of the vagina now, as it spreads open, _____, softening and yielding easily, easily around your baby as it descends . . . resting in between each and every contraction, coming to terms with becoming a mother now, being a mother now, can feel good, feels good to know the baby's coming down, down, to be cradled into your arms now, _____, into your arms now, the hips that used to cradle become the arms that cradle now, from hips to arms, from hips to arms, hands want to caress and *touch* your baby, your arms want to hold, to carry your baby on the outside. . . .

And you can feel the baby sliding down your vagina, almost like a slide that you might have slid down, _____, again remember the slide and the *glide* down that slide again and again. . . . And someone there to help you, to help you to be sure it's safe for you, _____, to slide and *glide* . . . you can feel that you want to let go, and you let go and right down you slide, down you *slide* to the very bottom, feels so good. You can, _____, remember the feeling of letting go at the top . . . just as you learned how to swing on a swing as a child and you learned how to let go, to glide through the air with the help of gravity on your side, now. Just as your baby's diving down your vagina, with the help of gravity, now. . . .

To personalize. **You may use the swing metaphor to stimulate the sensation of safely letting go with the help of gravity if it fits for you. Or you may insert your own metaphor based on a personal experience that simulates these same sensations of letting go, safely trusting gravity. Sensations based on your personal experience are the most powerful you can use. They will stay with you and be readily available during your labor.**

Second-Stage Labor And you can *feel* the contractions, coming and going, going and coming, each one gathering momentum as you push and your baby, _____, dives down with each and every contraction . . . you can feel yourself beginning to push and *push* and you can *feel* your baby diving down down, *down.* . . . It feels so good to your baby now, like an invigorating massage as your baby dives through your vagina . . . slipping and sliding down, slipping and *gliding* downward on the inside. . . .

And you can, _____, remember the sound of my voice, and my voice can go with you on the waves of each contraction, my voice can carry you . . . help you through each and every contraction, bringing your baby down.

Making Family And the voice of a husband or a friend can carry you down on the inside, can help meet the baby now, _____, greet your baby, resting in between each and every contraction, coming to terms with your baby now, coming to terms with anything that needs to settle in, settle in, now before the birth. . . . This is a very *flexible* time right now, as your body adjusts and adapts to the hormones that guide you through contractions. . . . Anything that needs a certain settling to help you feel that everything is in place for you . . . can occur . . . spontaneously as your baby settles

deeper and deeper down inside you, _____,
as if you are creating a settlement in a way . . . a safe and
secure settling into family. You can, _____,
feel the baby guiding you into family now.

To personalize. **Use your partner's name and the names of labor
assistants or friends who will be present at the birth. Also include any suggestions that reflect your experience in making a
family. Refer to your birth inventory for your specific concerns.
This may include fitting another child into the family and the
development of satisfying sibling relationships, especially if
sibling relationships were problematic in your childhood. An
example of a positive metaphor for sibling adjustment might
be the welcoming of another kitten into a litter, emphasizing
how kittens adjust, adapt, and snuggle together from birth. Develop your own metaphor as needed for your specific family
situation and write it in the space provided.**

_____

_____

_____

_____

_____

_____

_____

Then another contraction's coming, guiding you into
that basket of family, right for you now, _____,
a beautifully woven basket completely ready, completing
itself in ways that might even delight or surprise you as
you get closer and closer to your baby being born. . . . But
then another contraction is coming and going and going
and coming, always crashes and splashes, and releasing and
bringing the baby down so that you can hold your baby in
your arms *soon.*

And with the next contraction, _____, you   **Crowning**
begin to *feel* the baby's head, right down on your perineum.
You can feel the opening of your vagina begin to stretch,
burn slightly as you begin to *pant* and *pant* and your vaginal
opening stretches around your baby's head, now. And your
baby dives, can feel the wave building and building as you
pant . . . and pant and the wave builds and builds as the

baby's head crowns. But then the wave comes to shore, splashes to shore and you rest and your baby rests sinking deeper down, resting completely in between the contractions, now.

Birth You can feel your baby's head, can even put your hand right down and can feel that baby has hair on its head, can feel that hair now. But then another contraction is coming, and you can, _____, *feel* the wave surging and *surging*. Your baby wants to *see* you, *wants* to be born and you begin to *pant* and *pant* and you can *feel* your vagina opening and adapting and stretching right around your baby's head . . . and out comes your baby's head, right between your legs, and you can reach down to hold your baby's head, guiding it out with your own hands if you like. . . .

But then another contraction is coming, _____, and your baby's shoulders turn inside of you now as your baby slides, *glides* and you pant and pant and right out slip the baby's shoulders, right out slip its little knees and feet and toes, right out of your body now. A baby right into your arms, now that's where it's headed, right into your arms. Take your baby into your arms. Cradling your baby on the outside now, _____, where you can *meet* your baby!

Give yourself the right to hold that picture now . . . to see your baby in your arms now, looking down, down, down looking at those eyes looking up, up, up at you . . . little feet moving, little arms, moving in the air now. Can feel the baby against your skin. That's where it's headed, right next to your skin now. Can feel it right next to your breast. You can, _____, *touch* the baby's head with your hand now. Its little forehead relaxes under your fingertips . . . as you look down at your baby now. . . . And when you're ready . . . see your baby in another's arms, perhaps your partner, your husband, or your friend, or a dear relative holding that baby, holding that baby next to you now . . . and you can, _____, *look* at that person's eyes looking down and *welcoming* this little member of your family. . . .

To personalize. **Insert the person's name who will be holding your baby soon after birth, perhaps the father, a relative, or close friend. Also include a sibling holding the new sister or brother in his or her lap, with help if necessary. Write your suggestion in the space provided.**

_____

_____

_____

_____

_____

_____

_____

_____

_____

And now, _____, your family is whole, complete for now. As if you have woven the basket full, and the pear has dropped down to the earth and the flowers have opened with time . . . all in good time. And as you hold your baby close, or see your husband lovingly greeting your new baby . . . the wonder of it all can enter your heart now . . . and as you feel your heart full and waiting . . . you can let that scene slowly fade its way into your future, now. Feel the scene fade into the future, the near future where it belongs . . . surely awaiting you.

And remember, _____, that your baby, _____, knows full well the way out into your arms . . . just as your body knows how to complete the process of birth with a final contraction . . . a contraction you can look forward to, like a period on the end of a sentence, a caboose on the end of a train. This contraction doesn't hurt at all. The placenta is malleable, and right out plops the placenta full and whole. You can look at it later, if you'd like. . . . Your uterus will continue to contract sure and hard with your baby in your arms, down to its pre-pregnant size with time. . . .

Let that scene fade into the near future now, where it belongs, taking yourself back back back through the time tunnel, back into the womb now on the count of 10 back-

Remember the Placenta

ward, giving yourself time to *9*, skip *8*, *7*, right *6*, and *5*, falling slightly backward in time *4*, *3* you're getting *2*, ready *1*, to meet your baby on the inside. And take yourself inside the womb now, very, very deep inside, _____, you can feel your baby full, getting just a bit fuller, just ripe, just right for coming down. Dreams can help you, friends can help you, become ready as you become due. You are, _____, getting ready to become a mother. Yet you are *already* mothering on the inside in your pregnancy.

And with your next breath, _____, you can feel the baby on the inside, heavy and moving down, just getting ready, getting ready for labor, for birth. And give yourself the right to enjoy these last weeks of pregnancy . . . truly *enjoy* the last weeks and days you will look back on in the years ahead as the time just before meeting your child. . . .

Centering   And just centering yourself, _____, with your breath now, sensing how far you are from the walls, the ceiling of the room, from my voice, other people, feeling yourself as the very center of the room. And as the center becoming very ready, very energized, coming back to present time, to the sound of my voice, the temperature in the room, the sounds of your environment . . . adjusting and adapting as you bring yourself to a comfortable sitting position . . . taking this relaxation with you into the day.

Note to the mother. **This concludes a basic outline of the normal labor and delivery process. If there are situations that are not addressed in this outline, please alter it to fit your individual circumstances. This is your visualization! Make it work for you.** *And most of all, follow your journey, wherever it takes you.*

Adjusting to the Labor Process   Visualizing your birth will help you to become comfortable with labor when it occurs, no matter where your labor takes you. Whether you have a vaginal delivery, as imagined, or a cesarean birth, you have followed your baby. This is your job in labor—to follow your baby, adjusting to the labor process. Using the above tape will allow you to relax and enjoy the usual progression of labor. Should your labor take you down a different path, you will find the metaphors useful in dealing with contractions. The suggestions given will help you adjust in a more relaxed manner to whatever situation comes up. Greater resources for adaptation will make themselves available to you as the personalized suggestions put to rest distractions from your family history that might otherwise intrude.

Your personalized relaxation tape addresses your unique concerns about family adjustment and birth history, allowing you to work through feelings associated with childbirth and contributing to a decrease of tension and fear during labor.

Use the tape as often as you like for relaxation purposes. Once a week is minimal, and once a day is the maximum for women in my practice. You can also think of the tape as an experience unto itself, which may help you to resolve any loss from a previous childbirth. You may also use your tape to calm yourself if you feel anxious during the final month of pregnancy. Visualization has been found effective for facing and releasing fears and calming the spirit. Visualization can free your energy for easier adjustment to labor and can increase the potential for a healthy childbirth.

Your visualization also serves to open your heart to your child, establishing a bond before birth. And now that you have met your baby through your mind's inner eye, you can turn your attention to the days and weeks following the arrival of this new family member!

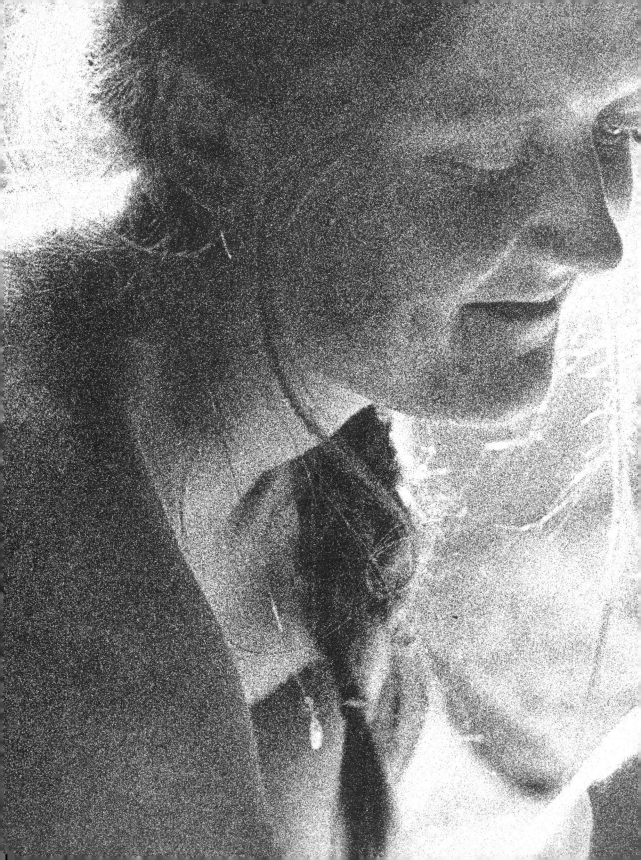

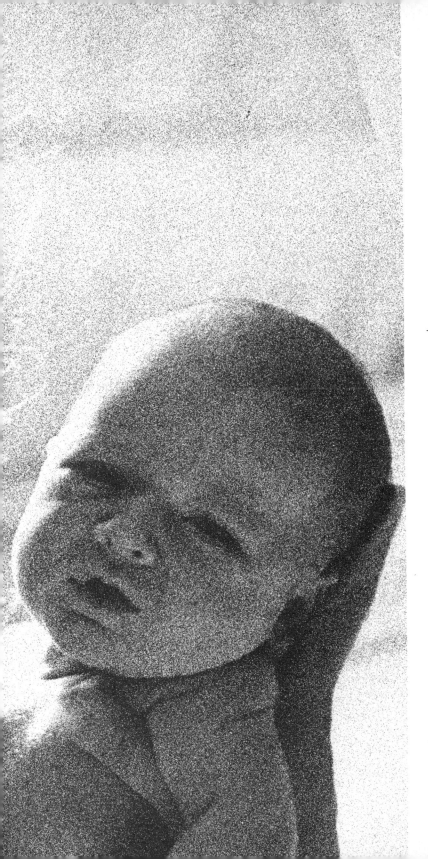

9

Bonding
with
Your Baby

*I never felt as close to my husband
as the night our newborn daughter
slept in his arms.*

JAMIE
on the birth of Rania

SOME MOTHERS AND FATHERS report an instant love affair with their baby from the moment of birth. Other parents need a period of acquaintance with their newborns before they feel a true bond develop. Whatever your immediate feelings are, rest assured that it takes time to know your baby. Your love will deepen naturally as you get to know this new little person.

Research by John Kennell and Marshall Klaus has shown that the first minutes and days after birth are critical periods for establishing a relationship with your newborn. It is equally important to realize, however, that you may need time to feel close to your baby. Although having your baby with you continuously, or as soon as possible, after birth contributes to family bonding, getting to know one another continues throughout your lifetimes together.

Meeting Your Baby

Ideally, both parents will be present when your child is born. Take time to smell, touch, and look at your new baby immediately, or as soon as possible after birth. Skin-to-skin contact with your newborn contributes to closeness and bonding. Take time to talk and share feelings with your partner as you acquaint yourself with your new baby. Watching your baby's adjustment together in the first hours and days after birth helps establish a very special beginning that you can share with your child when he or she is older. Children love to hear the story of their birth, their first meeting with you, and the weeks that followed. You are making history; you are making family. Enjoy it and remember it for the future. It becomes your family's folklore.

Telling Your Child's Story

In the space provided, write the story of your child's birth, including the first time you saw her or him, what your baby looked like to you, when you first held your baby, when you first had the impulse to kiss him or her, when Dad first held and kissed his child, other relatives' first meeting, and so forth.

_____

_____

_____

_____

_____
_____
_____
_____
_____
_____
_____
_____
_____
_____
_____
_____
_____
_____

Save this story and add to it later if you wish. Recording these impressions helps you capture your first few days with your baby—something to share with your child later when he or she can talk, listen, and play the game "Mommy tell me about when I was a baby...."

Physical Touch and Family Bonding

Newborns have a primary need for physical touching and stimulation. The first few days of life are important for skin-to-skin contact with your baby. If you are breast-feeding, this will happen automatically. If you are bottle-feeding your baby, however, you may need to take special time for physical touch. Fathers, too, benefit from skin-to-skin contact with their young. Holding your unclothed baby close to your naked chest is a warm and comforting welcome for a newborn.

In the days and weeks ahead you will get to know your baby and how he or she responds to the world. Some babies develop visually at first: Colors attract them, and they follow you with their eyes. Others are sensitive to sound: Noises arouse their interest, and they will turn to the sound of your voice. Still others are kinesthetically oriented and are sensitive to changes in temperature. These babies will often fuss more quickly for a diaper change. Your appreciation of your baby's personality will grow over time. These are the first few days of life, and these days are a special time for family bonding. Enjoy them. They are days you will remember forever.

Working after the Birth   You will adjust to the new family constellation, but it does take time to develop your relationships. Plan to have enough unscheduled time after birth to simply hang out together.

Both paternal and maternal leave from work are encouraged in many countries, including Sweden and Holland. Even though national policy in the United States does not support families in this way, you can make bonding your own priority after birth. Make arrangements to reserve a minimum of two weeks after delivery for family bonding and reorganization. One month is optimal. Both fathers and mothers should have time together with family as the major focus. Remember, the birth of this child happens only once. Time taken now for family bonding will ease adjustment in the months and years ahead. Do not let anxiety about money override the importance of this first month. Money can be borrowed and made up in the course of a lifetime. Its lack should not preclude your taking valuable time off at this critical point in your family's development. Time lost in getting to know your baby during the month after birth is time that can never be recovered.

Avoid any prearranged schedule for the first several weeks. You and your baby will develop your own timing as you get to know one another. A schedule will evolve naturally around the needs of all family members within six weeks or so. Allow your body to adjust to postpartum changes. Get plenty of rest and stay well-nourished.

Breast-feeding?   Research supports breast-feeding as the healthiest way to feed your baby, both physically and emotionally. It is also important, however, to consider each mother/infant relationship separately. If for any reason you have difficulty with breast-feeding, take your needs seriously. Seek help from your pediatrician and a breast-feeding counselor.

If difficulty persists, seek out a therapist for discussion of any emotional issues that seem pertinent. Visualization can be helpful here, too. Medical research has shown that imagery and relaxation techniques can increase milk supply in nursing mothers. There are also times when bottle-feeding can improve your mothering experience. What is most important is a happy and healthy relationship. Like other life situations, flexibility is the best approach. There are no hard and fast rules on how to love your baby. Seek help and discover what works for you and your baby. Feeding should be enjoyable for both of you.

Fathers are important to their newborns. At birth, babies can already recognize and respond to the paternal voice pattern. Psychiatrist Daniel Stern believes that infants are selectively attuned to both Father and Mother. Preliminary research by psychotherapist Bruce Linton suggests that infants have an inborn receptor for paternal/infant bonding. Dad is not merely a replacement for Mom; rather, fathers play a primary nurturing role to their newborn child.

Fathers Are Nurturers, Too

When mothers are not able to stay with their babies immediately after delivery, a father's presence can provide the security and warmth necessary while Mom recovers. Discuss this with your partner and make plans together so that one of you is there to welcome the baby in the event of a cesarean or other medical need.

Circumcising a boy child is no longer routine; it is a question with which many modern-day parents struggle. Dr. Benjamin Spock himself recently reversed his opinion on circumcision, stating at the Second International Symposium on Circumcision in 1991: "My own preference, if I had the good fortune to have another son, would be to leave his little penis alone."

Circumcision

Circumcision is no longer viewed as necessary for good health. The American Academy of Pediatrics reports that there is no absolute medical indication for its routine practice. Moreover, circumcision is painful to babies, particularly under the usual circumstances of hospital protocol. There are, however, reasons why parents still entertain the option of circumcision.

Religious considerations remain important. Some parents worry about the boy's likeness to other males in the family. These are the most common reasons that parents cite for choosing circumcision. There are no right or wrong answers; only you and your partner can decide what is right for your baby. In order to avoid regrets, however, it is important that the two of you discuss circumcision, and that you are both aware of your reasons for and against the procedure. It is important to come to a decision with which you both feel comfortable. This may be one of your first mutual decisions as parents.

If you decide on circumcision, it is advisable that you be present with your baby during the procedure. Emotional comfort before, during, and after the operation is important for your newborn. Babies who are held immediately before and after tend to cry less. If your child fell down and scraped his knee, you would hold him as he cried, and he would feel better because of it. Circumcision is the same. Your baby will feel better if he experiences your warmth and comfort.

In the traditional Jewish *bris*, relatives, friends, and family are present to witness and celebrate the circumcision as part of a covenant with God. Some parents report that during this ritual their baby scarcely cried. The *bris* takes place eight days after birth instead of in the first day or two after delivery, as is common in the hospital setting. This passage of time allows your baby to adjust to the change of being outside of the womb, and it gives family bonding time to develop. If you decide to circumcise, use common-sense guidelines for comfort and timing of the operation. Your son will benefit from the loving consideration of his parents.

Relatives Grandmothers and other relatives may be helpful in the days following delivery, depending on the nature of your relationship. Be aware that relatives may also welcome feedback regarding what kind of help you need from them and what you wish to do on your own. There is no substitute for learning about your baby yourself, with the support and love of others nearby. Let others help you, if desired, but express yourself freely if relatives try to take over in ways that inhibit your own discovery of parenthood.

Children between the ages of two and five, and even older, may revert to more dependent behavior after the birth of a sibling. Three-year-olds may want to return to their bottles instead of drinking out of cups. Some may even want to wear diapers again. Ordinarily, this is a request for reassurance that you are adding a child to the family, not replacing one. Patience and a little extra nurturance from Mom, Dad, and other relatives can contribute to feelings of security.

Older Children and Regression

Reserving some special time with the older child is important. The amount of time is less crucial than the quality of time spent together in an activity that the older child can enjoy. It is also important that the activity be something an older child can enjoy but that babies are too young to appreciate. Acknowledge your youngster's feelings verbally and stress the advantages of being older. Reading a story together, for example, can give the child special attention while at the same time reinforcing the message that special privileges and abilities come with growing up. Babies, after all, cannot enjoy or even understand stories—because they are not old enough. Babies' needs are important too, but they are different.

Some regressive behavior will disappear within the first month to six weeks after birth. Within four months, most siblings show affection toward the baby and resume age-appropriate behavior. If for any reason intense jealousy persists beyond this time, especially if the child shows no signs of developing affection toward the baby, it may prove fruitful to consult a family counselor. Getting the help you need when you need it is the key to healthy family adjustment.

Include siblings as much as possible in family activity and bonding during the days immediately following birth. This allows older children to adjust and begin their own relationship with their little brother or sister. Pointing out to older children how they can help, as well as the advantages they have that babies do not yet enjoy (like eating ice cream), helps the child feel not only loved but also proud.

Older Children Adjusting to a New Baby

There is a natural interest and curiosity that babies show

for their older siblings. Point this out. Explaining to your older child that the baby has a special look for older sister or brother encourages this special bond.

It is important to keep changes to a minimum during the first three months after the birth of a new sibling. This reassures the child that his own place in the family is still secure. For example, major changes in day-care arrangements following the birth of a younger sibling can strain the older child's relationship to the newborn. Children are less likely to associate loss of attention from Mother or Father with rejection if they are not sent away to a new place and new people when baby arrives on the scene.

Be sure that any day-care arrangements are in place for at least six weeks before the birth. Establishing and adjusting to a new day-care situation well before baby arrives allows the older child to adapt to one change at a time. Even if the day-care schedule changes later, returning to an established day-care relationship and environment during this sensitive period reduces the possibility that your child will feel overwhelmed by new people and places.

After the initial excitement wears off, most older siblings will become bored with the new baby and want to return to activities with children their own age. The key is that your child already have these external relationships in place. This allows for a smoother family adjustment during the months after birth—with less possibility of establishing patterns that will evoke future sibling rivalry.

Postpartum Blues and Support   The amount of family adjustment required during the year following birth is greatly underestimated. Motherhood may come easily to you, yet changes are inevitable and must be accommodated. Hormonal fluctuations can increase emotional sensitivity, but the feelings that arise are real responses to real changes—both physical and emotional.

Postpartum blues are common during the three months after childbirth. Mild sadness may well up as your body recovers from pregnancy and delivery and you adjust to the life changes that having a baby can bring. Isolation is the main cause of acute depression. Support groups for new parents can help you make contacts for babysitting and answer some of your needs for companionship. More important, a new-parents support group can banish the misunderstanding that motherhood is instinctual. It is not. Mothering is very much a learned experience. Much of what we know about it is learned unconsciously, relayed to us during childhood by those who cared for us.

The Myth of the Mothering Instinct

If we were held and cuddled in a loving and reassuring manner as infants, we automatically know how to do that with our own babies. Our bodies hold the knowledge, so we experience it as instinct. If you did not receive confident mothering in the arms of your own mother, you may find yourself unsure.

If this happens, you can establish a network of other mothers from whom you can learn now. Learning from others with a variety of childhood experience will help you understand your own needs. This is a prime time to find a healthy balance between your needs and your baby's needs.

Visualization for Bonding with Your Baby

This exercise can help you to gain perspective and get in touch with any past blockages that keep you from enjoyment of your baby. Refer back to your own blueprints for parenting in chapter 2. In the space provided, write down what, if anything, was missing from your own early experience of being mothered.

_____

_____

_____

_____

_____

_____

_____

_____

_____

_____

_____

_____

_____

_____

_____

Take time to identify feelings that might come up for you during the postpartum period. Visualize yourself as a baby, getting whatever it is that you needed. More holding, more secure cuddles, kisses on the cheek, being talked to softly —absorb these images fully. You may want to include your partner—even have him hold you in his arms—or share the exercise with a friend who can nurture and comfort you.

Then, after you have taken these moments for yourself, imagine your baby smiling up at you—looking cute and cuddly—and feel your love for your own child, growing with time, as you learn to love and care for this baby, too: getting to know each other, laughter and tears bonding you together now. You are remembering that time passes, seeing your child grow in your mind's inner eye—to three years, seven years, ten years, then to teenage years, sixteen years, eighteen years . . . to adulthood. A time of sharing seems so long but as you adjust to your baby, you will be amazed at how fast babies grow and how soon you will be watching yours leave home . . . to continue the cycle of life.

By gaining a perspective on your own childhood, with the help of a support group, a family counselor, or a friend, you can find what will help you nourish both yourself and your baby at the same time. Do not ignore these needs. If you get help now, your enjoyment of parenting will greatly increase. You deserve to enjoy your baby!

Within the first year after birth, most mothers experience complete adjustment to the new family constellation. Postpartum blues usually resolve within three months after delivery. Occasionally women experience severe depression, which must be professionally treated. Get whatever help you need. How you respond to your own needs and those of other family members forms the foundation for your family relationships.

Bonding after an Emergency Delivery

When babies have been separated from their mothers and fathers after birth due to medical intervention or other complications, they are sometimes extra sensitive to noises, strangers, or sudden changes in the environment. For days or weeks following birth these babies may be more irritable and fussy. They may be reacting to early deprivation.

These babies, as well as their mothers, may need special attention and loving care. In my work with women and their babies, I have discovered that emotional separation after birth, especially for a prolonged period, may trap both mother and baby in a loop of negative feedback. I believe that in such cases both mother and baby are in some way reliving the birth experience, unable to resolve the pain of early separation. When this is the case, simply taking time to heal the experience through visualization while the mother holds her baby, can calm them both. It can also create a positive change in their relationship. The following case illustrates the problem of oversensitivity resulting from emergency procedures at birth, and one way it can be resolved.

Alice delivered her daughter, Emma, by cesarean section due to distress during labor. Emma was taken by ambulance to another hospital immediately after birth. Emma's father stayed with Alice, so Emma was without family members around her until the following day, twelve hours after being born, at which time her father went to see her. Following observation and medical examination it was determined that Emma was, in fact, fine. She was returned to her mother three days after birth.

When Alice came to see me, two months after her baby's birth, she could not relax and appeared very nervous about her ability to care for Emma. She reported that she answered Emma's every cry, sometimes crying with her for hours at a time when she could not quiet or comfort her. She loved her baby very much but was having an extremely difficult postpartum adjustment since Emma, who was rarely quiet and contented, usually screamed even when held. Alice had consulted with her pediatrician, who could find no physical reason for Emma's excessive irritability and heightened sensitivity.

I observed during the session that Emma startled and cried very suddenly and very loudly at almost every change in the environment. Her cries were piercing and frantic—unlike most babies, whose cries are usually shorter and who are more easily comforted.

As we reviewed her birth experience, Emma began to wail frantically. Alice said this was her usual behavior. I pointed out that the experience of being in a strange place and in strange hands during the days after birth may have made Emma particularly needy, and that Alice was, in fact, doing a wonderful job of mothering Emma through this unusual beginning. I suggested that Alice go back to the birth and imagine what it would have felt like to have held Emma in her arms immediately after birth. After all, she had missed this, but it did not stop her from being able to hold her now and imagine what her wish could have been for herself and for her baby.

Speaking over Emma's frantic screams, I instructed Alice to breathe and to relax, holding Emma close. I suggested she imagine the birth as she would have wished it to be and simply enjoy visualizing herself holding Emma and keeping her close after birth. She knew now that Emma was fine, and she could take that knowledge back with her to the time of birth, allowing it to change the picture back then, healing the past—holding her close and warm, no separation at all, just keeping her next to her after she was born. . . .

Within two minutes of visualizing and relaxing into a healing visualization of this imagery of bonding after birth, Emma abruptly—as abruptly as she had begun—stopped crying and looked around the room and at me for the first time. Alice and I continued to talk about the possibility that Emma had developed an overwhelming negative and fearful response to any change in her environment, however slight, based on her first experience of being whisked off in an ambulance with sirens blaring and no one to hold or comfort her through the many medical procedures she endured in the hours that followed. What a shocking way to enter the world! We also talked about the healing visualization, the feelings of holding Emma immediately after birth with no separation, and giving herself this healing experience now and throughout the next few weeks. Later in the session, Emma cried again, but much more quietly, and she responded to Alice's holding—and imagery of holding her after the birth—by becoming quiet.

The most striking part of this story is the fact that from that day on, Emma's crying spells tapered off, soon becoming normal. She became consolable, and Alice's relationship with her baby was free to develop without undue strain. By the following month they were not only loving, but also enjoying one another.

I believe that some babies and mothers may find themselves in a negative-feedback loop after a very negative or difficult delivery experience. If it is not resolved, the baby may re-experience fear based on early trauma, which reactivates the mother's own trauma and unresolved emotions about the birth. These feelings are passed from one to the other in subtle body movements and tension. Women who have been separated from their babies due to medical emergencies often experience guilt and pain, which is reflected in how they hold their babies. I believe the healing visualization helped Alice and her baby reconnect in a new and different way.

You may wish to construct your own images for healing if you feel your relationship with your baby is suffering unnecessarily because of feelings surrounding the birth. Usually this takes the form of an excessively irritable baby who is particularly sensitive to changes in the environment and reacts negatively and fearfully. The baby is usually difficult to console.

Visualization for Distress at Birth

By allowing yourself to go back and visualize the experience as you would have liked it, paying particular attention to those moments when you wanted to hold your baby, or be alert and present, you change the movements of your body. Your touch will now communicate feelings of confidence rather than uncertainty. Babies do feel connected through your body, and feelings are physical. Healing visualization can affect your feelings, and your touch will soon impart calm and reassurance.

If you feel that you and/or your baby may have felt fear during labor, birth, or immediately afterward, and you believe it is inhibiting a positive relationship, go back to visualize the experience as you would have wished it to be. First, visualize it by yourself. Identify what you needed or wanted. Then, share it with your partner or a friend. If you wish, you can have someone help you visualize a change by repeating phrases to you that feel healing, such as seeing yourself hold your baby right after birth, taking your knowledge that your baby is safe and healthy back to a time when you had fear, holding that younger you who was afraid during or after the birth. . . . Use whatever images work for you. Write them in the space provided.

_____

_____

_____

_____

_____

_____

_____

_____

_____

_____

_____

_____

_____

_____

_____

_____

_____

_____

_____

_____

_____

_____

_____

_____

_____

_____

_____

_____

_____

_____

_____

When you feel ready, close your eyes and visualize these images while holding your baby. Feel the contentment, healing, and love of these images communicated to your baby through your body, heart, and mind. This should take only three to five minutes. Then set the images aside, and continue to enjoy your baby.

These images and feelings will remain with you and can help you feel calmer and more confident in your mothering as time goes on. Your baby will respond to your experience.

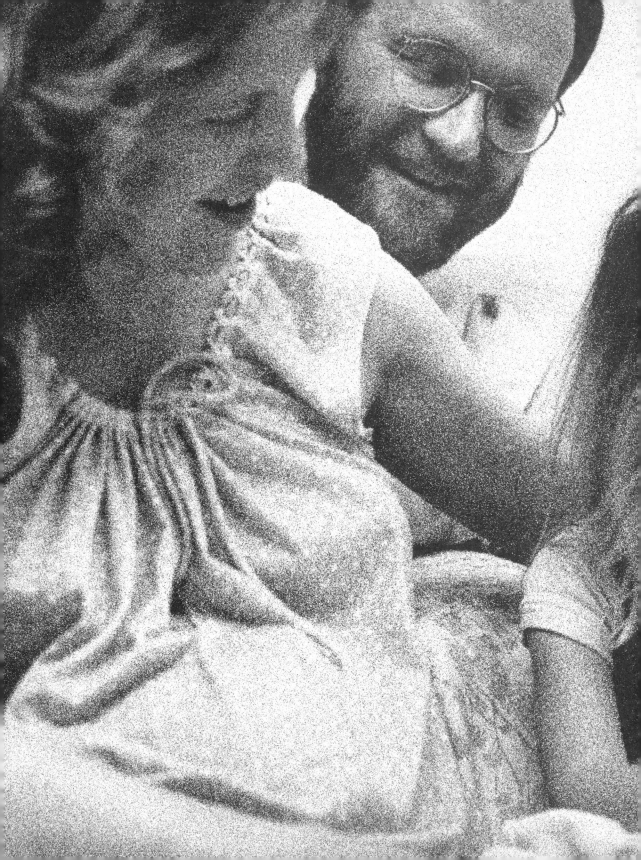

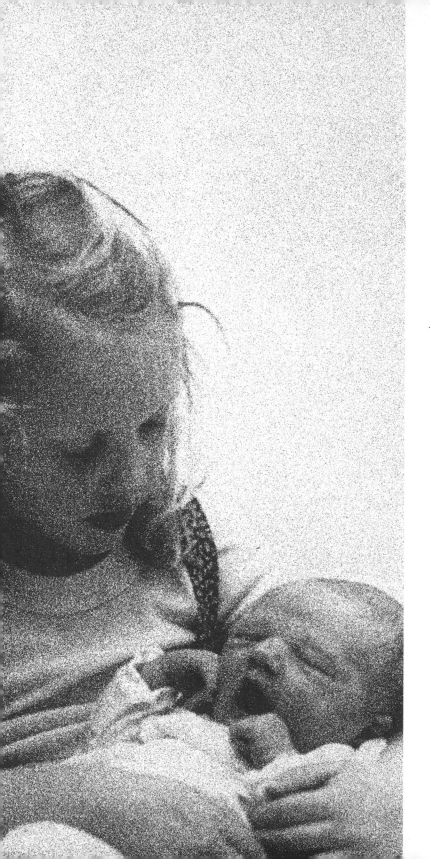

10

Becoming a Family

*I believe in loving and being loved
. . . without loving and being
loved, the human soul and spirit
would curdle and die.*

VIRGINIA SATIR
Peoplemaking

THE BIRTH OF A BABY is the birth of family. Myriad births take place at once: Women become mothers, husbands become fathers, daughters become sisters, and sons become brothers. One birth ripples through generations, creating subtle shifts and rearrangements in the family web. The first year following the birth of a child is a time of great, and often underestimated, adjustment. How you begin relationships during this period can influence your family's future.

Together, you and your partner can create either greater fulfillment or increased tensions in your lives together. Your awareness of your family as a whole that is greater than the sum of its parts is important if you and your partner are to balance successfully the needs of all family members, including your own.

The first year of life is a time to establish healthy family relationships and interactions. The way you nurture your newborn and the manner in which you support each other as parents will stay with you throughout your family life together. It will also influence the relationship between the two of you. In this chapter we will focus on the development of healthy family relationships during the postpartum period.

Your Couple's Bond

One of the main tasks of families is to raise and nurture children to adulthood. The family is the garden in which individual members grow and develop. The health of the garden depends to a great degree on the nature of the couple's bond. If parents can give loving support to one another, they can teach the values of nurturance. Children benefit and grow from living with parents who feel loved and supported by each other.

If you give consistent love and nurturance to your child, but you allow your relationship to become a desert, your child senses the lack of the love between you, even though he or she can't articulate the feeling. Instead, children become more needy, demanding more of what is missing but not defined. This causes unnecessary strain on your family. Your child will feel loved and learn how to love by watching your relationship with each other. Therefore, it is important to set time aside for yourselves. Babies flourish not only from your direct attention but also from the love you give to each other.

Talk to each other about your relationship. Your relationship deepens as you share life and time together. Sharing now allows you to know each other better. Talking about feelings deepens your relationship as parents and as partners.

Planning Time Together

Plan on a dinner out or a walk together as a couple within three months after your baby arrives. Find a person you feel safe and comfortable leaving your baby with for one and one-half to two hours. By the time your baby is three months old you have begun to establish a routine. The two hours you take may be a time your baby naps. Or your baby can enjoy a relative or a reliable friend while the two of you take some time just to be together. Your baby will benefit from the time you focus on one another. You can look forward to the feeling of being alone together after your baby is born. New life experience can deepen your relationship if you are communicating. Sharing feelings now can create a new kind of intimacy.

Sexuality and Intimacy

For three to four weeks following birth, while a mother makes her physical recovery, it is necessary to abstain from sexual intercourse. For some women, a drop in estrogen levels and the challenges of motherhood can affect sexual drive for up to a year following birth.

Many women feel less interest in sex during the months following birth, especially if they are breast-feeding. Postpartum hormonal changes may thin vaginal tissue and lessen lubrication during intercourse. Sexual drive will return naturally if the relationship with your partner remains intimate. It is important that partners not perceive reduced sexuality as inadequacy or lack of love.

A woman's lessened sexual drive may also be caused by lack of energy. She is absorbed in nurturing the baby. When men take the opportunity to be primary emotional care givers they experience similar feelings. As tiredness diminishes, you will free up energy for other enjoyable activities with your partner, including sex.

It is important to discuss sexual feelings with your partner and not to mistake sexuality for intimacy. Sexuality may symbolize the desire for closeness, but it is not a substitute for talking. Communicating your needs and expressing your feelings to one another can bring you closer. Sexuality can be a form of communication and certainly an expression of love. If partners are miscommunicating or misunderstanding one another, however, sexual activity often fades. If partners are communicating their needs and feelings to one another, and taking time to discuss the changes they are undergoing, they become closer and more bonded. If they are coping with the changes through isolation and distance from one another, they drift apart, becoming lonely instead of intimate.

Occasionally, passion dies completely because of lack of attention to the relationship. Then, when a couple becomes physically ready for more sexual activity, they may not be close enough emotionally to ignite the spark. You can avoid this by staying in touch with one another. Plan regular dates and schedule time for your relationship.

Will Your Partner Feel Left Out?

Sometimes men feel lonely and left out of the emotional life of the family after the baby arrives. If fathers are included as primary nurturers in the family, this can be avoided. It is common, however, for men to feel that they are secondary, not only to their wives but also to their babies.

A support group for new and expectant fathers can provide a wonderful opportunity for working through feelings that fatherhood brings. Fathers can benefit from the support of other parents going through similar life changes as much as mothers can. Fathers need the support of other men to become fathers themselves, and women cannot provide that help. Find out what resources are available for men in your community. You can always start a group of your own.

Communication and a Successful Partnership

Parenting may feel instinctual, but it is learned behavior. Your own parents were your first role models, and each of you will have flashbacks to your own childhoods through parenthood. Some of these memories will evoke pleasure and give you confidence in your roles as parents and partners. Other memories will have negative or unpleasant associations you would rather forget. Don't! Painful memories will help you work through your fears and make it less likely that you will repeat your parents' mistakes.

Refer to chapter 2 again. Review the exercise concerning your own family backgrounds with your partner. By understanding your respective histories, you will be able to guide your own family in ways that you perceive as most beneficial. You will be better able to decide the kind of parents you want to be.

Father/Infant Relationship

Fathers must develop their own relationship with their newborn. A baby is more secure if it has more than one primary nurturing relationship. Sometimes fathers fail to develop their own relationship with their babies because the mother spends more time with the baby. As time goes on, the mother, being quicker to intuit the baby's needs, becomes the prime nurturer—even when the father is present. This often leaves the father further and further behind as the family develops, and he eventually becomes peripheral to its life. The mother/infant relationship tightens. The father's feelings of being outside the mother/child bond grows. And the couple's relationship withers.

One guideline to keep in mind during the first months after birth is that the person spending the most time with the baby will react to the baby's needs sooner. Usually this is the mother. It can be helpful to remember that your husband can and will develop his own relationship with his baby, and it will be different and separate from your own.

A father needs time alone with his newborn to develop his own style of caretaking. He needs to learn how to comfort, diaper, and nurture his child in his own way. It's natural for Dad to take more time to understand exactly what the baby may need and how to comfort him or her, if he has not been spending as much time with the baby as Mom. Do not mistake this for an inability to care for the baby. Babies and fathers can work out their own relationship together.

Don't interfere if you see your partner struggle with the diaper or display awkwardness holding the baby. Like you, he needs time to learn. Interrupting this learning disrupts father/infant bonding. Instead, support this relationship by leaving Dad with his infant for a period of time. By one month after birth, even nursing babies can be left with Dad for a minimum of two hours while you take time for yourself. Your baby will not starve, and Dad will learn how to provide primary nurturing to his young son or daughter. Bonding deepens as people learn together. To lessen their struggle is to decrease their opportunity to develop a connection.

Developing the Father/Child Bond

In the space provided, write a few sentences about baby's first time alone with Dad. How did Dad care for his baby? How was this different from how Mom does it? Did they have fun together? What special bond do they have together?

_____

_____

_____

_____

_____

_____

_____

_____

Healthy Family Relationships

Research on family systems psychology began in the 1950s and has come a long way in identifying what contributes to healthy self-esteem. This is a wonderful time to be a parent because we can benefit from new knowledge about the characteristics and communication styles that create healthy families. Nurturing self-esteem is the foundation for family love and caring.

Remember that you are growing together and making your own family. You can make new rules and change old patterns; it doesn't have to be exactly like the family either of you came from. Sort out what was good and nurturing from your past and be aware of what you wish to change. If you need support, talk with a counselor or a friend, or join a support group with other parents who are having similar experiences.

You have just completed a part of your emotional preparation for pregnancy, birth, and the postpartum period. The rest will come with experience. Working through this book has put you in touch with important challenges in family life that lie ahead. If you have followed the exercises, you have developed several resources: inner reflection; self-nurturance; plus the ability to identify your needs, communicate them to others, and get the support you need. These have become your tools for a period of growth and change. This new knowledge of yourself will help you develop your own inner resources for labor and birth and more importantly, for life.

You are at the beginning of an adventure in family making. Happy birthing! And remember that the changes you make now will be passed on to your grandchildren.

1

Case Study—
The Peterson Method

THE FOLLOWING EXAMPLE WILL help you to understand how the exercises in this workbook can help you.

past childbirth

Terri came to see me in her sixth month of pregnancy for preparation for her second childbirth. Her first baby had been born after a difficult and prolonged labor resulting in forceps delivery. Terri was twenty-seven at the time. She remembered that he had been in a posterior position, and that his head had not presented correctly. The impact of Sean's birth left Terri with a distinct fear of loss of control. She was also anxious about her body's ability to give birth at age thirty-nine. We met three times. Our sessions lasted two hours and were scheduled once monthly during her last trimester.

*fear of giving birth
at thirty-nine*

Terri very much wanted a baby and was willing to put aside an established career to stay home and nurture her child. She had been married to her second husband for eight years and enjoyed a stable and loving relationship. They were both looking forward to having a baby and had

normal ambivalence

planned the conception. Nevertheless, she still felt ambivalent. Terri's ambivalence was normal, much like that of many modern women who are faced with integrating career, motherhood, and new family relationship.

Terri worked to clarify her feelings about her first childbirth experience and to identify instinctual feelings associated to her childhood. She also acknowledged worry that

fears related to sibling rivalry

her older son might see the new baby as an intruder. After all, he had never had to share his mother with a sibling before. He had enjoyed the attention of being an only child.

feelings of loss and abandonment during childhood and early motherhood

She also expressed some concern that her husband might leave her. This feeling stemmed in part from an abandonment experienced in her family of origin when her father became increasingly emotionally distant from her, culminating in what Terri described as estrangement when she was thirteen and her sixth sister was born. As the eldest of seven children, Terri was overburdened with taking care of her younger siblings while lacking the loving attention she needed. She had also divorced her first husband when her son was three years old, leaving her with the emotional belief that having babies and marriage did not agree. Her fear of losing control during labor and of suffering a recur-

negative childbirth experience

rence of the terror of her first childbirth was clearly entangled with her family history of loss and abandonment.

When Terri visited her midwife the day before her labor began, she was told that this baby was in a posterior position, as her first son had been. She was warned to expect a slow labor. Afterward she sent me the following letter

personalized birth visualization tape

describing the birth. In it she refers to phrases used during the birth visualization that we had taped for her.

> . . . and so straight down and out he came in a two-hour labor. The day before he had been posterior, and my midwife remarked that because of this, my labor would be slow. On December 1st at 3:30 p.m. my plug broke. I took a hot bath and drank warm milk thinking the baby would be born sometime this weekend. Around 6 a.m. I listened to the birth visualization we had taped during our last session . . . there was lots of activity from Eliot. Around 8 a.m. my labor kicked in and at 9:55 a.m. he was born . . . bright and beautiful!

Terri had worked to resolve the fear of her first birth during which her baby did not present correctly. Certainly for Terri, the change to normal presentation and the unexpectedly rapid two-hour labor serves to confirm that she gained a sense of mastery by talking about the feelings associated with her first childbirth, and then listening to suggestions that included "This baby coming straight down on your cervix, straight down and out." This suggestion had been repeated several times on her preparation tape.

clearing previous childbirth

Terri's letter continued:

Throughout the pregnancy, labor and now one week later, different phrases you had said float in my mind. Also wonderful has been the sweet bonding between the four of us.

The suggestion for bonding between the four of them had been included on Terri's birth preparation tape, which she listened to during her last month of pregnancy. We had included this suggestion because it was an important concern for her throughout her pregnancy, and it addressed her anxiety specific to this childbirth.

Terri's preparation also included a realistic approach to the pain of labor and she was able to identify her personal strategies for dealing with labor:

identifying coping strategies

I used low gutteral sounds and squeezed my husband's hand to handle contractions. It helped so much to be in relationship to my labor rather than so afraid. . . .

Terri discovered that her natural coping style was kinesthetic. Her strategy of squeezing her husband's hand released tension and pain through her abdomen. Free of fear, Terri had more energy available to cope effectively with contractions.

During our work together, Terri acknowledged many concerns related to childbirth, unearthing anxieties that otherwise might have absorbed energy needed for labor. Terri faced the shadow side of her decision to have a baby, resulting in a deeper commitment to her unborn child. Expressing her fears readied her for motherhood. This left her with an abundance of energy with which to approach labor and her new baby:

During pregnancy, labor and now new motherhood I needed to go inside to find my courage, strength and inspiration. . . . Oh, I know adjustments will continue . . . but I am amazed and happy at the sweetness of it all.

Summary The following list is an inventory of the issues that Terri addressed during her prenatal preparation:

1. Fear of a repetition of the complicated birth of her first child
2. Anxiety about being thirty-nine at the time of her second childbirth
3. Concern about how she would blend an established career and the needs of a newborn
4. Concern about how her twelve-year-old son would accept a younger sibling
5. Associations of the loss and emotional abandonment she felt in her strained relationship with her father and as a new mother when she divorced her first husband
6. Fear of losing control during labor and an inability to cope with or manage the pain

During our six hours together Terri shared her fears about the upcoming labor and recognized her anxieties about new motherhood. Expression of these concerns brought her both comfort and the ability to visualize family bonding. She recognized her natural coping style for pain and learned realistic methods for confronting her next labor. She was able to separate her prior difficulty in childbirth and the abandonment in her former family relationships from her current pregnancy and family. This allowed Terri to ask for what she needed and gave her a sense of mastery and readiness for birth and new motherhood.

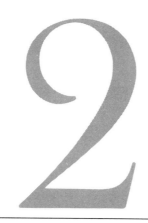

Transforming Fear

THE FOLLOWING EXERCISE IS one therapists commonly use to help patients deal with a particular fear. By facing your fear you will be better able to transform it to a useful learning experience. Naming your fear is the first major step to its resolution.

What are your fears about labor? When you imagine yourself in labor, are there any fears or anxieties that seem particularly significant? Look slowly and carefully at this inner picture of yourself. Write down any fear or concern that you feel needs your attention at this time. You may want to refer to your birth inventory.

_____

_____

_____

_____

_____

_____

_____

_____

_____

_____

Now take out some crayons or other drawing material and several sheets of paper at least twelve by fifteen inches to give yourself plenty of room to draw a picture, design, or simple shapes and lines that describe the fear. Draw different fears separately or express them all in one drawing; use color and shapes to symbolize your fear and remember: This is not a test of your artistic ability but an opportunity to externalize fear. You may choose to show this picture to your partner, a supportive friend, or a therapist if you are currently working with a professional. Describe what is in your drawing to this other person. What do you dislike most about it? Is there anything about it you like or could use constructively? Is there anything you could learn from the fear? What do you need to help you resolve this fear?

Now take a few minutes to identify what you would like to change about this drawing. What would give you a better feeling about it? How can you transform the fears expressed in your drawing? How would it feel to have mastered the fear, bringing yourself to a place of safety and power? Now draw that picture! Use all the colors available to express this new feeling. Use one paper or many. Then describe what you have drawn to the person with whom you have chosen to share your fear and its resolution. Tell this person about anything you may have learned about yourself from this exercise.

Fear is a natural human response, but it is not one that need stop you from your own development. This exercise can help you make friends with your fears and look past them for what you want and need for yourself. Before you transform the fear, you must name it. This exercise can help you face your fear and release energy for dealing with labor and birth. It did so for Jenny, as described in art therapist Nora Swan-Foster's essay "Images of Pregnant Women" (reprinted from *The Arts in Psychotherapy*, vol. 16, pp. 283–292, Pergamon Press, 1989):

Jenny was thirty years old in her sixth month of pregnancy. She had recently remarried. Her pregnancy was going well but she experienced intense imagery and emotions concerning her

first pregnancy, which had been complicated by vaginal herpes
and resulted in cesarean birth. She wanted her second pregnancy to be a vaginal childbirth experience.

When she was asked to draw a picture of her fear, Jenny
sighed and slowly drew a zigzag in the upper left hand corner
and described it as the "nee" feeling of herpes. She described
herself as the blue airy line looking up at the doctor holding a
knife. She described the red sun symbol with the yellow center
and rays coming out from it as her fear that her current husband
would not be able to support her just as her first husband had
not supported her. The triangle and square represented her
jobs. When Jenny finished drawing she said,

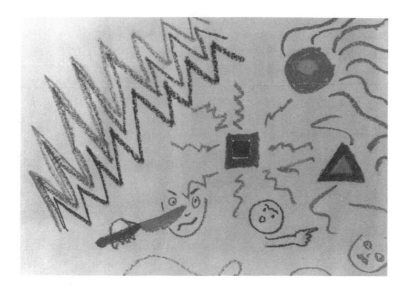

'The knife is coming into the craziness and stress and cutting
me open. And it brings up the fear that I'm just going to be
passive and a nonentity, powerless, and people will be making
decisions, crowding me, and then cutting me. After I drew this
I saw all the stuff between me and my husband and how I'm
not protected in this drawing.'

By acknowledging her fears and feelings, Jenny was beginning to put her past behind her while defining her needs that
would support her desired childbirth experience. This process
of separating out the past from the present was making room
for a fresh childbirth experience and a new baby.

In her second drawing, Jenny imagined how she would transform the fears expressed in her first drawing. As she drew she laughed and said,

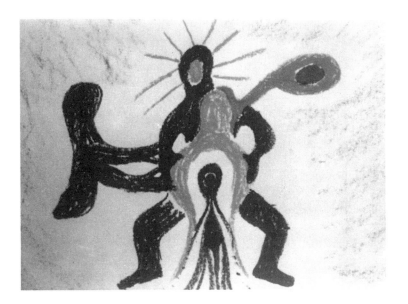

'This is me giving birth. I started with the lighter, center image—it's open, very open. The darker images in the middle of and extending out of the light figure are the baby in the uterus. The person with yellow rays behind me is my husband supporting me. He looks like the Hulk, Spiderman—he looks strong. The oval symbol on the right in blue is a support person or something cool and relaxing and the figure on the left is the midwife, but of course I'm the main character during birth. The shading around all of this is God—this drawing feels extremely strong.'

Jenny decided to use this second drawing as a positive image of strength and power to replace the old imagery of weakness and loss. She gave birth vaginally, expressing how much the drawing had helped her heal the past so she could be free to imagine a more positive outcome. Jenny found images which empowered her as a woman.

Should feelings arise that are particularly bothersome to you and that remain with you after the exercise, you may want to consult a professional therapist for counseling.

When physical ailments arise during pregnancy, we seek the counsel of an experienced medical professional. It is important to rely on ourselves, to trust our bodies and not run to the physician for every twinge or pain we feel. There are times, however, when it is a sign of health to reach out to an expert who can help you respond to emotions that feel overwhelming or particularly difficult. More and more people are getting the help they need from support groups, family therapy, and other mental health services. As the field of mental health loses its stigma, more people are paying attention to their needs and feelings—turning away from their addictions or painful patterns to live healthier and more productive lives.

3

A Review of the Natural Flow of Labor

Effacement to About Four Centimeters Dilation

First Stage: Early Labor

The thinning and early dilation of the cervix may take from five hours to twenty-four hours or more. Some of the thinning happens without your awareness, during what is sometimes referred to as the latent phase of labor.

Signs of labor starting include a bloody show, regular contractions, or breaking of waters. With subsequent babies, this early stage may be hard to delineate. Keep in mind that labor is a part of the process of pregnancy and may not be experienced in well-defined stages but rather as an expression of energy evolving outward.

Slow breathing may help you stay calm and centered. Walking, sewing, reading, cooking, or other early-labor projects and relaxing activities are important now. Eat if you are hungry; you will need the energy. Keep track of your liquid consumption; be sure to empty your bladder regularly—at least every thirty minutes—particularly if you are drinking a lot of fluids. This will prevent an overly full bladder, which could cause unnecessary pain and possibly slow the labor.

First Stage: Active Labor   *Four to Eight Centimeters Dilation*
Contractions are strong and closer together, lasting longer; these are effective in opening the cervix, which is by now fully effaced. Walking and other activity usually is no longer comfortable, particularly if this is your first baby.

Slow, deep breathing may be used in combination with vocalization or other coping techniques. Relaxing between contractions is important now. Your partner may do well to remind you to let go of tension between contractions. Visualize the cervix opening wider and wider, as the baby's head comes through.

So-called Transitional Stage   *Eight to Ten Centimeters Dilation*
No significant change delineates this part of active labor, other than increased intensity. The same coping techniques you've been using continue to be useful. Continued heavy labor; contractions may become longer and be somewhat irregular. These are some of the longest and most intense contractions you will experience. The sensation of an impending bowel movement is normal as the head begins coming through your cervix toward the vaginal canal. Backache, nausea, irritability, and sweating profusely are reported by some women. Others, however, experience only a steady augmentation of intensity. You will be completely immersed in the activity of labor by now and would probably do well to concentrate on the tremendous power coming through you, consciously directing energy through your body and out your vagina. Visualize your vagina as stretching open and the contractions traveling through you to open the way for your baby. Remember to continue breathing.

Bloody show may occur, if it didn't earlier, as well as breaking of the waters. Deep breathing in combination with panting to avoid early pushing may be useful now.

The Baby Travels through the Birth Canal   **Second Stage of Labor**

The feeling of bearing down or pushing involuntarily along with spontaneous vocalization or grunting during contractions are common now. The baby's head will be seen from the outside but will slip back at the end of a contraction until crowning. Your vagina will be massaging your baby at this point, getting it stimulated for breathing. A burning sensation may be felt around the outside of your vaginal opening with each of these contractions as the baby moves outward and then retreats. Panting can be a very useful technique to prevent pushing and thus allow the vaginal opening to stretch slowly around the baby's head without tearing. Perineal massage and support may be helpful here. Visualize the vagina stretching open for the baby's head. Let it happen. After the baby's head is out, another contraction or two may be needed to birth the rest of the baby's body. This is normal.

Expulsion of the Placenta   **Third Stage**

Any time between five and forty-five minutes after birth you will feel another contraction, which will expel the placenta. This usually feels good and almost never hurts. Putting the baby to your breast to nurse may help stimulate this contraction. Afterward, the nurse, doctor, or midwife may suggest that you gently knead the uterus down so that it feels like a hard grapefruit. This is good to do after birth and intermittently for the next twenty-four hours. Contractions will be felt for about four to five days after birth as the uterus returns to its pre-pregnant size. The most effective remedy for the discomfort of afterbirth contractions is massage and gentle holding by your partner. Emotional support is a great pain reliever. Use it.

If you desire, ask that the placenta be put aside so you can look at it later. It is a detailed and fascinating organ. Many women turn their fascination to the placenta after initial engrossment in the baby, only to find that it was disposed of before they had a chance to see it.

4

Physical Exercise

EXERCISE IS IMPORTANT to your emotional and physical health. Pregnancy is no exception. Aerobic exercise is necessary for keeping the cardiovascular system in good shape for labor. In terms of energy expenditure, labor has been compared to a fifty-mile hike. The following exercises should be done daily and are primarily aimed at limbering and strengthening muscles for an easier labor and birthing. They should not, however, be used as a substitute for general exercise, such as yoga, walking, dancing, and tennis. They should be done in addition to your normal activities.

This is only a brief guide to get you started. Refer to *Essential Exercises for the Childbearing Year*, by Elizabeth Noble, for a thorough approach to exercise during pregnancy and descriptions of positions that might be useful during labor.

Kegels: Relax, as when urinating, then contract the pelvic floor muscles as if to stop the flow. Hold this muscle contraction to the count of twenty to one hundred, then release. The duration of the hold is more important than the number of repetitions. Do at least five per day.

Squat: For a minimum of five minutes per day take a squatting position. Squat whenever it is convenient throughout the day as well.

Cat stretch: Squat, then move into hands-and-knees position. Contract buttocks down toward the floor and inward, tipping the pelvis, letting head and shoulders drop down toward hips. Then reverse the stretch by swaying the back sticking the buttocks out, and neck and head up toward the ceiling. Do complete stretch at least four times daily. This is particularly good for backaches and relieves pressure on internal organs during pregnancy.

Leg stretches: Sit in tailor fashion with soles of feet together. Use hands to push the knees toward the floor, gently increasing the stretch to the inner thigh. Do this for five minutes daily.

Leg pushes: Lie flat on back, knees together, legs bent with soles of feet flat on the floor. Partner places hand on outside of knees and exerts steady pressure while woman slowly presses knees apart to the count of five. Then reverse, partner places hands on inside of knees exerting steady pressure while woman brings knees together to the count of five. This is an isometric exercise.

Stretch and relax position: Sit on the soles of your feet, legs folded, thighs at right angles. Rest hand by your sides, palms facing back. Head leans forward until forehead rests on floor. Turn head to either side and rest in that position. Relax. Do this once daily; hold as long as comfortable. Get used to being able to get into this position as it is sometimes used during labor to dilate a cervix with an anterior lip (the term used when the front of the cervix dilates more slowly than the rest of the cervix).

Concentration: Practice holding the gaze of your partner eye to eye for three minutes. Laughter is common the first several times you do this exercise, but practice will make it a tool for use during labor. It can help you make or reestablish contact with one another.

BIBLIOGRAPHY

Arms, Suzanne. *Immaculate Deception*. New York: Bantam, **Books**
1977.

Balaskas, Janet. *Natural Pregnancy*. New York: Interlink,
1990.

————. *The New Active Birth*. London: Unwin, 1989.

Bettelheim, Bruno. *A Good Enough Parent*. New York:
Knopf, 1987.

Bing, Elisabeth, and Libby Coleman. *Having a Baby After
Thirty*. New York: Noonday, 1989.

Boston Women's Health Book Collective. *Our Bodies, Ourselves*. New York: Simon & Schuster, 1971.

————. *Ourselves and Our Children*. New York: Random
House, 1981.

Brewer, Gail, and Tom Brewer. *What Every Pregnant Woman
Should Know: The Truth about Diet and Drugs in Pregnancy*.
New York: Penguin, 1985.

Chamberlain, David. *Babies Remember Birth*. New York: Bal-
lantine, 1990.

Cohen, Nancy. *Silent Knife*. South Hadley, Mass.: Bergin
& Garvey, 1983.

Davis, Elizabeth. *Hearts and Hands: A Midwive's Guide to
Pregnancy and Birth*. Berkeley, Calif.: Celestial Arts, 1987.

DelliQuadri, Lyn, and Kati Breckenville. *The New Mother
Care*. Los Angeles: Tarcher, 1984.

Deutche, Helena. *The Psychology of Women*. New York:
Grune and Stratton, 1945.

Dick-Read, Grantly. *Childbirth without Fear*. New York: Harper & Row, 1944.

Donovan, Bonnie. *The Cesarean Birth Experience*. Boston:
Beacon Hill Press, 1977.

Fedor-Freybergh, Vanessa, and V. Vogel, eds. *Prenatal and
Perinatal Psychology and Medicine*. Park Ridge, New Jer-
sey: Parthenon, 1988.

Gibran, Kahlil. *The Prophet*. Alfred Knopf, New York. 1923.

Gilligan, Carol. *In a Different Voice*. Cambridge, Mass.: Har-
vard University Press, 1982.

Greenberg, Martin. *The Birth of a Father*. New York: Avon,
1986.

Grinder, John, and Richard Bandler. *The Structure of Magic*,
vols. 1, 2. Palo Alto, Calif.: Science and Behavior Books,
1976.

Hampden-Turner, Charles. *Maps of the Mind*. New York: Macmillan, 1981.

Hathaway, Jay, and Margie Hathaway. *Children at Birth*. Sherman Oaks, Calif.: Academy, 1978.

Hilgard, Ernest, and J. Hilgard, eds. *Hypnosis in the Relief of Pain*. Los Altos, Calif.: William Kaufman, 1975.

Jordan, Brigitte. *Birth in Four Cultures*. Montreal: Eden Press, 1980.

Kitzinger, Sheila. *The Complete Book of Pregnancy and Childbirth*. New York: Alfred Knopf, 1980.

———. *The Experience of Childbirth*. New York: Pelican, 1981.

———. *Being Born*. New York: Grosset & Dunlap, 1986.

———. *Breastfeeding Your Baby*. New York: Alfred Knopf, 1988.

Klaus, Marshall and John Kennell. *Parent-Infant Bonding*. St. Louis: C.V. Mosby, 1980.

Lamaze, Fernand. *Painless Childbirth*. New York: Pocket Books, 1959.

Lang, Raven. *The Birth Book*. Fulton, Calif.: New Genesis Press, 1977.

McGoldrick, Monica, and Elizabeth Carter, eds. *The Changing Family Life Cycle: A Framework for Family Therapy*. New York: Gardner Press, 1988.

Noble, Elizabeth. *Essential Exercises for the Childbearing Year*. Boston: Houghton-Mifflin, 1976.

———. *Childbirth with Insight*. Boston: Houghton-Miffling, 1983.

Peterson, Gayle. *Birthing Normally*. 2nd Ed. Berkeley, Calif.: Shadow and Light, 1984.

Peterson, Gayle, and Lewis Mehl. *Pregnancy as Healing*. Berkeley, Calif.: MindBody Press, 1984.

———. *Cesarean Birth: Risk and Culture*. Berkeley, Calif.: MindBody Press, 1985.

Panuthos, Claudia. *Transformation Through Birth*. South Hadley, Mass.: Bergin & Garvey, 1984.

Pryor, Karen. *Nursing Your Baby*. New York: Pocket Books, 1973.

Richards, Lynn Baptiste. *The Vaginal Birth After Cesarean Experience*. South Hadley, Mass.: Bergin & Garvey, 1987.

Rossi, Ernest. *The Psychobiology of Mind-Body Healing.* New York: W.W. Norton, 1988.

Satir, Virginia. *Peoplemaking.* Palo Alto, Calif.: Science and Behavior Books, 1972.

Stern, Daniel. *The Interpersonal World of the Infant.* Basic Books, New York, 1985.

Verny, Tom, and John Kelly. *The Secret Life of the Unborn Child.* New York: Summit Books, 1981.

Willson, Robert, Clayton Beecham, and Elsie Carrington. *Obstetrics and Gynecology.* St. Louis: C.V. Mosby, 1975.

American Academy of Pediatrics. *Circumcision.* Available from P.O. Box 1034, Evanston, Ill. 60204.

August, R.V. "Hypnosis in Obstetrics". Chapter 6 in *Hypnosis in the Relief of Pain* by Ernest R. Hilgard and Josephine R. Hilgard. New York: McGraw-Hill, 1961.

Bibring, Greta. "Some Considerations of the Psychological Process of Pregnancy." *Psychoanalytic Study of the Child* 14 (1959): 113–21.

Chamberlain, D. "The Significance of Birth Memories." *Pre- and Perinatal Psychology* 2 (1988):4.

Cheek, D. "Maladjustment Patterns Apparently Related to Imprinting at Birth." *The American Journal of Clinical Hypnosis* 18, no. 2 (1975): 75–82.

Crasilneck, H.B. and J.A. Hall. "Clinical Hypnosis in Problems of Pain." *American Journal of Clinical Hypnosis* 15 (1973): 153–61.

Davidson, J.A. "Assessment of the Value of Hypnosis in Labor." *British Medical Journal* 2, no. 5310 (1962): 951–53.

Davis-Floyd, Robbie. "The Technological Model of Birth." *Journal of American Folklore* 100 (1987): 398.

Feher, S., L. Berger, J. Johnson, and J. Wilde. "Increasing Milk Production for Premature Infants with a Relaxation/Imagery Audiotape." *Pediatrics* 83 (1989): 57–60.

Gorsuch, R.L., and M.K. Key. "Abnormality of Pregnancy as a Function of Anxiety and Life Stress." *Psychosomatic Medicine* 36 (1984): 352–62.

Hansen, John. "Older Maternal Age and Pregnancy Out-

Articles and Other Resources

come: A Review of the Literature." *Obstetrical and Gynecological Survey* 41 (1986).

Hodnett, Ellen, and Richard Osborn. "A Randomized Trial of the Effects of Monitrice Support During Labor: Mothers' Views Two to Four Weeks Postpartum." *Birth* 16 (1989): 4.

Kennell, J.H., M.A. Trause, and M.H. Klaus. "Evidence for a Sensitive Period in the Human Mother." In *Parent-Infant Interaction* (Amsterdam: CIBA Foundation Symposium 33, New Series, ASP, 1975).

Klaus, M.H., R. Jerauld, N. Kreger, N. McAlpine, M. Steffa, and J.H. Kennell. "Maternal Attachment: Importance of the First Postpartum Days." *New England Journal of Medicine* 286 (1972): 460–63.

Lederman, E., B.A. Lederman, and J. Work. "The Relationship of Maternal Anxiety, Plasma Catecholamines, and Plasma Cortisol to Progress in Labor." *American Journal of Obstetrics and Gynecology* 132 (1978): 495.

Levenson, G. and S. Shnider. (1979). "Catecholamines: The Effects of Maternal Fear and Its Treatment on Uterine Dysfunction and Circulation." *Birth and Family Journal* 6, no. 3 (1979): 167–74.

Lindberg, Cheryl, and Frank Lawlis. "The Effectiveness of Imagery as a Childbirth Preparatory Technique." *Journal of Mental Imagery* 12 (1988): 103–14.

Linton, Bruce. "Developmental Stages of Fatherhood." Unpublished Manuscript, 1991.

MacDonald, M., M. Gunther, and A. Christakes. "Relations Between Maternal Anxiety and Obstetrical Complications." *Psychosomatic Medicine* 25 (1963): 74–77.

Mehl, Lewis, Gayle Peterson, Nancy Shaw, and Donald Creevy. "Complications of Home Delivery: Report of a Series of 287 Deliveries in Santa Cruz County, California." *Birth* 2 (1975): 123–25.

Mehl, Lewis, Gayle Peterson, Louis Leavitt, and Donald Creevy. "Comparison Study of Home and Hospital Birth." *Proceedings of the Fifth International Congress of Psychosomatic Obstetrics and Gynecology.* New York: Harper & Row, 1976.

Mehl, Lewis, Carol Brendsel, and Gayle Peterson (at the Institute for Childbirth and Family Research). "Children at Birth: Effects and Implications." *Journal of Sex and Marital Therapy* 4, no. 3 (1977).

Mehl, Lewis, Gayle Peterson, and Louis Leavitt. "The Relation of the Home Birth Movement to Medicine and Psychiatry." *World Journal of Psychosynthesis*, 1979.

Mehl, Lewis, Gayle Peterson, and Carol Brendsel. "Personality Variables and Labor." *Birth and Psychology Bulletin* 1 (1') (1979).

———. "Episiotomies and Pelvic Floor Symptoms." *Women and Health*, 1980.

Mehl, Lewis, and Gayle Peterson. "Evaluation of Non-Nurse Midwives." *Women and Health*, 1980.

———. "Home vs. Hospital Birth: A Matched Comparison Study." In *Pregnancy, Birth, and Parenting: Coping with Medical Issues*, edited by P. Ahmed. New York: Elsevier-North Holland, 1981.

———. "Existential Risk Factor Screening." In *Pregnancy, Birth, and Parenting*, edited by P. Ahmed. New York: Elsevier-North Holland, 1981.

———. "Parent-Child Psychology: Delivery Alternatives." *Women and Health*, fall, 1987.

Mehl, Lewis, Jo McRae, Laura Grimes, and Gayle Peterson. "Phenomonological Risk Screening for Childbirth: Successful Prospective Differentiation of Risk for Medically Low-Risk Mothers." *Journal of Nurse Midwifery* 28 no. 5 (Sept./Oct. 1983).

Mehl, Lewis, Sharon Donovan, and Gayle Peterson. "The Role of Hypnotherapy in Facilitating Normal Birth." In *Prenatal and Perinatal Psychology and Medicine*, edited by P. Freyburgh, and M.L. Vanessa-Vogel. Park Ridge, N.J.: Parthenon, 1988.

Omer, H., D. Friedlander, and Z. Palti. "Hypnotic Relaxation in the Treatment of Premature Labor." *Psychosomatic Medicine* 48, no. 5 (1986).

Peterson, Gayle. "The Effects of Childbirth on Women's Self-Esteem." Paper presented at the 13th Annual Meeting of the Psychological Association, Toronto, 1976.

———. "Addressing Complications in the Prenatal Setting." *Journal of Nurse Midwifery* 28, no. 2 (March/April 1983).

———. "Prenatal Bonding, Prenatal Communication, and

the Prevention of Prematurity." *Pre- and Perinatal Psychology* 2, no. 2 (1987).

———. "The Emotional Aspects of Prenatal Care." In *The Ultimate Guide to Health and Fitness*, edited by Cynthia Riddle. Topanga, Calif.: Vortex Publications, 1988.

———. "The Peterson Method for Body-Centered Hypnosis in Childbirth." In *The Encyclopedia of Childbirth*, edited by B. Rothman. Phoenix: Oryx Press, 1991.

Peterson, Gayle, and Lewis Mehl. "Some Determinants of Maternal Attachment." *American Journal of Psychiatry* 135 no. 10 (Oct. 1978).

———. "Psychological Outcome Studies of Delivery Alternatives." In *Freedom of Choice in Childbirth*, edited by D. Steward and L. Stewart. Marble Hill, Mo.: NAPSAC Press, 1979.

———. "Beliefs, Attitudes, and Birth." *Mothering*, spring 1985.

Peterson, Gayle, Lewis Mehl, and P.H. Leiderman. "The Role of Some Birth Related Variables in Father Attachment." *American Journal of Orthopsychiatry* 49 (1979).

Peterson, Gayle, Lewis Mehl, and Jo McRae. "Relationship of Psychiatric Diagnosis, Defenses, Anxiety, and Stress with Birth Complications. In *Prenatal and Perinatal Psychology and Medicine*, edited by P. Freyburgh and M.L. Vanessa-Vogel. Park Ridge, N.J.: Parthenon, 1988.

Poncelet, Noelle. "An Ericksonian Approach to Childbirth." In *Ericksonian Psychotherapy, Volume II, Clinical Applications*, edited by Jeffrey Zeig. New York: Brunner-Mazel, 1985.

Sosa, Roberto, John Kennell, Marshall Klaus, Steven Robertson, and Juan Urrutia. "The Effects of a Supportive Companion on Perinatal Problems, Length of Labor, and Maternal-Infant Interaction." *New England Journal of Medicine* 303, no. 11 (1980).

Swan-Foster, Nora. "Images of Pregnant Women: Art Therapy as a Tool for Transformation." *The Arts in Psychotherapy* 16 (1989): 283–92.

Videotapes, Audiotapes, and Slides

Arms, Suzanne. *Dania's Birth* slides of a family-centered labor and childbirth, available from Suzanne Arms, Cornell St., Palo Alto, Calif.

Hartigan, Harriette. *The Birth Disc*, a visual documentary of the childbirth process and additional slide series of birth also available through Artemis, 3337 McComb Ave., Ann Arbor, Mich. 48108.

Informed Birth and Parenting. *Special Delivery*, a 40-minute videotape about three women's labors. Available from Informed Birth & Parenting, P.O. Box 3675, Ann Arbor, Mich. 48106.

Noble, Elizabeth, and Leo Sorger, M.D. *Channel for a New Life*. A 40-minute videotape of an outdoor waterbirth. Available from Elizabeth Noble, 448 Pleasant Lake Avenue, Harwich, Mass. 02645.

Peterson, Gayle. *Body-Centered Hypnosis for Childbirth*. A 60-minute training videotape for professionals. Available from Shadow & Light Productions, 1749 Vine St., Berkeley, Calif. 94703.

————. *Pregnancy, Birth and Bonding*. A 90-minute audiocassette tape for pregnant women, using body-centered hypnosis for prenatal bonding and childbirth preparation. Available from Shadow & Light Productions, 1749 Vine St., Berkeley, Calif. 94703.

Yotvat, Iris. *Nine Moons*. A 40-minute videotape of one woman's preparation for vaginal birth after Cesarean. Available from Injoy Productions, 1490 Riverside Rd., Boulder, Co. 80304.

Organizations

Cesarean Prevention Society
P.O. Box 152
Syracuse, N.Y. 13210

Informed Homebirth
P.O. Box 3675
Ann Arbor, Mich. 48106

International Childbirth
Education Association
P.O. Box 20048
Minneapolis, Minn. 55420

LaLeche League
9616 Minneapolis Dr.
Franklin Park, Ill. 60131

National Association
of Childbirth Assistants
205 Copco Lane
San Jose, Calif. 95123